WITHIN NORMAL LIMITS
"WnL"

MARCO ANTONIO GAMBOA

WITHIN NORMAL LIMITS
"WnL"

Halo
PUBLISHING
INTERNATIONAL

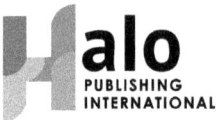

Halo
PUBLISHING
INTERNATIONAL

Halo Publishing International
7550 WIH-10 #800, PMB 2069,
San Antonio, TX 78229

First Edition, October 2023
ISBN: 978-1-63765-495-8
Library of Congress Control Number: 2023917423

The story presented in this book is entirely a product of the author's imagination
and is purely fictional. Any resemblance to actual persons, whether living or
deceased, or actual events is purely coincidental.

Halo Publishing International is a self-publishing company that publishes adult
fiction and non-fiction, children's literature, self-help, spiritual, and faith-based
books. We continually strive to help authors reach their publishing goals and
provide many different services that help them do so. We do not publish books
that are deemed to be politically, religiously, or socially disrespectful, or books
that are sexually provocative, including erotica. Halo reserves the right to refuse
publication of any manuscript if it is deemed not to be in line with our principles.
Do you have a book idea you would like us to consider publishing? Please visit
www.halopublishing.com for more information.

To Penelope
and Adalaide

Preface

This entire book is fictitious in the most extreme sense of the word. It was written slowly between 2013 and 2023. The book was born from having two children, marrying and divorcing twice, losing touch with the love of my life, being diagnosed with multiple sclerosis, and living on a street where a murder-suicide occurred.

Sitting for most of those ten years in isolation, pain, dizziness, confusion, and often convinced by others I had lost my mind, I wrote these stories.

In fact, I write this preface to you half naked from the floor of my bedroom. Alone in a four-bedroom house, with strong doses of medications intended to lull the pain and calm my muscles; however, they are also attacking my ability to be mobile, stay awake, and understand reality.

But this is where the book came from, because as I eventually float towards a very familiar and comforting Vantablackesque haze, I pray as best I can that I dream of my girls, Colorado, or the backyard I cannot currently get to.

Thank you for reading.

Marco

Contents

CHAPTER 1

The Mother's Unforgiving Reality

The man wailed as if he were knowingly being torn away from life, inch by inch, flesh by flesh.

The students facilitating the demo ran to console him.

His left arm went numb during the stroke he had twelve years before, but now, as the medical students walk up to unplug his virtual reality set and the pads wired to his arms, legs, and chest, the man throws his numb arm in all directions with every intent of punishing everyone around him.

"No," he screamed.

"No, no, no," he pleaded. His begging fluctuated from that of a man being thrown off the edge of a planet, to that of a child being left by the soul of a parent.

"Please."

"Please turn it back on."

"Please."

With one of the swings he took at the students, he fell out of his chair.

His mother, who had driven him to the lab and had been outside getting coffee, ran in at the sound of her son's voice.

"Just ten minutes. Just ten seconds. Give me my body back. Give me my mind back. Let me feel happy. Let me keep myself company."

No one tried to get him up off the floor.

The stoic professor watched his students more than he watched the man who on the floor. He knew some might stop the program, as this would be the first of a lifetime of occurrences of their watching someone hopeless, and in return it would diminish their hope. This was their first time to understand that their best intentions might still leave them hopeless. And even when attempting to mute the haunting of past, present, and future patients, no fine dinner, no extravagant vacation, no time with friends, and no time with family would ever allow them to forget the pleas of those in pain.

The mother crouched beside him. The man was forty-seven; the mother, sixty-eight.

"Mom," he whispered.

His voice, to her, was still childlike, and this hurt her. It was the voice of a child afraid of the dark, one always first to run out of the elementary school and straight into her arms.

"Mom?"

"Honey, what happened?"

"Mom, they made it go away. But now it's back, Mom."

"Made what go away?"

"All of it," he said. "I was me."

The mother looked at the professor.

"Ma'am, I'm so sorry; like the disclosures you signed stated, this is a trial of the equipment, and there will be kinks we must work out."

The virtual reality (VR) sets and wires attached to sticky pads were meant to recreate the visual, physical, and emotional effects of multiple sclerosis, so the medical students could experience the disease through wearing them. But with the man, during the calibration process, the machine began to establish a baseline, and it made the disease vanish for him, instead of projecting the disease onto the students.

In short, the man had experienced a moment of not having multiple sclerosis, not having had the stroke, and not carrying the weight of all the memories tied to each. The pain and fear he'd carried for more than twenty years had vanished momentarily.

"Mom, I want to go home."

The mother looked up towards one of the other volunteer patients.

"What's your name?"

"Marco."

"Marco, help me, please, get him in his chair."

"Sure, but can a couple of you help too? My balance is off today," he asked the other volunteers.

Two women got up, and they all walked over to the man who lay motionless on the floor and helped him into his chair.

As the chair embraced him and the present moment continued to suffocate him, he let out a defeated cry.

The mother strapped his upper torso to the chair with a seat belt.

"Please, five more minutes," he pleaded.

The mother reached behind the wheelchair, clicked a button to remove control of navigation from the man, and began to push him toward the door.

The whole thing had triggered a flare-up in him, and he was now slurring what sounded like additional pleas. The eye that was not paralyzed searched the room endlessly, looking for a place to rest or a face to help, but it never found one. Most of the students were looking down toward the ground. A few had quietly left through the exits in the back of the room.

As the mother exited the building, using her back to push the door open, the professor finally stood up. "I'm sorry," he said.

She gave him a half-blameful smile, nodded, and turned to the right of the exit once she had cleared the door.

CHAPTER 2

Marco's Journal Entry
June 2004

She was part of the staff who were newly hired for the summer. Even though I was only twenty-two, I was already an older member of the staff, and it was obvious she was a college kid home for the summer. I wondered where she was going to school. Was it somewhere exciting? Or somewhere just new, a place to reinvent yourself into someone more interesting?

My sister was like that, too. She thought living in a large city would make her more interesting. The sad thing was, she was already super interesting, but she just didn't see it. And if she didn't see it now, she'd never see it.

The bar was round, with chairs for guests all around. TVs hung in every corner of the area, so people could watch whatever games were on. To the side of the bar was the area for guests waiting for a spot in the bar or a spot on the other side of the restaurant for formal seating. Next to the waiting area was a huge glass that separated the waiting area from the kitchen. Families would often crowd the glass as they watched cooks grill and prepare their food. If there were a lot of kids, the cooks would throw butter on the grill and make enormous eruptions of fire that would warm the glass. They'd do the same, however, if there was an attractive woman watching.

I finished pouring the Long Island iced tea into the cold mug that I had carried instead of setting it down. My gaze fixated on a girl who was part of the new-hire group. At the moment, the cooks and waitstaff were all huddled together, getting in their pre-meal talk. The mug was hurting my hand, and I spilled quite a bit of the drink onto the bar counter. I handed the mug over to a man in a blue shirt. I cleaned up the spill with the last remaining towel that was stored behind the bar. When I looked up, I saw that the huddle had dispersed, and the entire group of new folks were standing around looking a little intimidated.

I wanted to go to the alley and try to talk to her. I was curious what her voice was like. I wanted to know what her eyes were like when she stared at me. I wanted to try to make her laugh. But at the moment, there was nothing that needed me in that area, and more people were walking up to the bar, looking around, trying to figure out which television was airing their game and which part of the bar was less sticky.

Just then, the man in blue said, "Let me get a cup of chili. This tea's going to hit a little too hard without anything in my stomach."

I nodded quickly and ran toward the kitchen. As I got closer, I could feel my heart pounding, both from running quickly and from the nerves brought on by possibly saying the wrong thing to her. I stopped running and walked quickly toward where the group was looking straight at the floor. As I neared the kitchen line, I yelled out for a cup of chili.

The yell alone, I knew, was enough to get her attention because it is human instinct to be alarmed by loud noises. She startled, and I smiled at her, and she at me. She was gorgeous, tall, and had light-brown hair that was up in a bun. She had hazel eyes and long, thin fingers. She wore the standard uniform of T-shirt and jeans with Chuck Taylor shoes, which were maroon. Her eyes wandered everywhere with a curiosity I envied for some reason.

My heart pounded as I was handed the chili, and I did all I could to not trip or drop the bowl. In recent years, I had become clumsy. I also was thinking constantly of my enunciation. I had been told that sometimes I slurred, which I attributed to being sleepy half the time. But I always responded that English was not my first language, and so I hid my accent and had to translate my thoughts, but that was usually an attempt to cover up that I knew I was soft-spoken.

We were now next to each other. She was examining the kitchen, and the kitchen crew had caught on. Like a bunch of hungry animals, they were already talking to her. "Sweetie, don't order food later. Just tell me what you want, and I'll cook it for you. I'll tell you what, just tell me what you don't like, and I'll make something just for you. We want you to feel welcome here," said the oldest line chef, the fucking savage.

She laughed and said okay.

Just as I was about to ask her what day she was working this week, the manager walked out and asked the new crew to come to the office to sign paperwork.

I had missed my chance. Back toward the bar and waiting area, it looked as if it was shaping up to be a full house. I grabbed the chili and headed toward the bar.

"You forgot the spoon, the crackers, the garnishes. C'mon, Marco," said the Love Chef.

The whole kitchen laughed.

"We'll see who forgets what when you guys get more than three tickets and panic," I quipped back.

We all laughed.

I ran back defeated to four people waiting to place an order and a machine holding three printed tickets.

As I walked up, Lindsay, my bartending partner for the evening, leaned toward me. "You're ugly as fuck, Marco," she said as she kissed my cheek. "I'll tend to the folks, and you work the machine."

I smiled. "Sure," I said.

Before the new girl, there was Lindsay, who was kind and had a great laugh, but who was also now engaged and pregnant with her first baby. My being late with women was often something that occurred. But I was invited to her wedding in Vegas after the baby was born, so there was that.

I walked up to the well area of the bar and pulled what were now six tickets from the machine. Two Budweisers, one Coors, four Shiners, and three Texas teas. What was interesting about the Texas tea was that when I was really busy, I sometimes forgot the tequila, but not once had anyone complained. Our teas in general were not for those who savored taste, but for those who savored the fuzzy clarity that came when liquor took the wheel and let us sit in the back seat or in the passenger seat and just watch the night sky pass above us. It was, and is, a beautiful thing.

"I'm your help tonight."

Looking down to avoid making a mess, I didn't recognize the voice. "That's racist," I said. "We've come a long way from that."

A boisterous laugh came, one that started with a very well-pronounced *B*. I looked up. It was she—the new girl.

"Hi, I'm Sarah."

"Hi, I'm Marco."

"But, for real, I was assigned to help the bar out tonight. No clue what that means, but here I am."

"It's actually pretty easy. You run food for us when it's ready in the expo area, and you run drinks, after I make them, to the tables."

"Deal."

"Where are you from?"

"I'm actually from here. I just graduated high school and need a job until I leave for college in August."

"That's exciting."

"I guess. I just want to live alone, and one college accepted me," she said, ending with a much smaller laugh.

I smiled. The printers immediately shot out ten more tickets.

"Let's do this. I'll start running these out." She grabbed all the beers and walked away. I watched her hair bounce and the curls extend as she turned and took a few steps.

Again, the loud laugh that made me daydream about a life in which that laugh was the only constant.

She stopped and turned around. "Where do I go?"

I laughed and said, "Look, each ticket has a table number and the order summary. The table numbers are actually etched on the sides of the tables, but if you look at the restaurant, they all go in order, starting back there with the tens, and over here with the eighties."

"Got it."

"If you feel comfortable with your balance, reach down under the bar over there. In the bar frame, there are trays you can use."

She laughed again, and I fell more in love. "I'd rather drop less at a time. I'm not taking more than these hands can carry."

I smiled, and the night began.

What I noticed was that anytime she walked near anyone, people noticed her. She always had a gaze that seemed the utmost interested in what anyone said. I knew she was going to make a lot of money and make me fall further in adoration.

The night was so busy we rarely spoke. But, each time we exchanged drinks, she'd make a comment—"Good job," "This one looks good," "If I was twenty-one, I'd ask you to make me one of these." Maybe she hated silence.

As the night died down for the restaurant, business was steady at the bar. There was a good game on, and a lot of the regulars had come around. She knew her facts about the Spurs and even predicted it back then; we were witnessing a dynasty.

Finally, she walked up, visibly exhausted, little sweat beads on her forehead, and her apron dusty with peanut-shell casings and salad-dressing stains. "The manager said that since it's dying down, I can leave."

"I had fun with you being the help."

She laughed—I had needed to make her laugh once more.

"I'd hang out, but I'm eighteen, and they know that. So it'd be weird if you served me."

"It would be, and I can't get fired, or else I won't be able to feed my five kids."

Her eyes widened. "Wow, that's exciting," she said in a staccato tempo.

I smiled. "I don't have kids. I don't even have a girlfriend."

"Maybe when I'm done with training, they'll let me be the waitress who works the bar area."

"Deal," I said.

"Okay, anything before I leave?"

"One last thing…huge favor. Our regulars just ordered a round of shots, and so I'm about to make those, but I have a customer who's been waiting for me to get him a bowl of Grandma's chicken noodle soup."

"I didn't know we had chicken noodle soup!"

"Yeah, it's an old menu item that only people who have frequented for a while know about. Truthfully, I think we're only carrying it until the frozen packs we have go bad. Go yell for it on the expo line, and tell them, after I finish my drinks, I'll ring it into the system to add it to the tab."

"Deal." She took off running.

I stared down toward the floor and closed my eyes.

The lobby was quiet enough to hear her say, "A bowl of Grandma's chicken noodle soup, please and thank you!"

I opened my eyes to see the kitchen guys smiling. The oldest walked over to her to clarify what she had just asked for. I saw her talking to them and pointing at me.

The entire kitchen and a few of the tenured folks erupted in laughter. Even the dishwasher, who usually communicated only in Spanish, came out to laugh. He held her hand, and I was told later that in broken English, he told her, "No chicken soup *aqui*, honey. Maybe next door."

I smiled and then laughed as I watched her walk back to me.

"MOR-TI-FIED. You get your own fucking soup next time."

I laughed.

Lindsay walked up. "See, Marco, you're ugly and an asshole. That never works out."

Sarah laughed. "Well, for sure an asshole." And then, "Night, guys," Sarah said as she walked away.

CHAPTER 3

The Evil the Strings Tell Us About

Gorecki was on the radio, and neither Linda nor her boy-friend, Ivan, knew who he was, nor that it was Symphony no. 3, op. 36. Had their neighbor, Marco, not been passed out from drinking, however, he would've known—he loved it. Particularly the part where the Virgin Mary speaks to her dying son on the cross, "My son, my chosen and beloved, share your wounds with your mother."

That's where Linda had heard it before, from Marco's blaring radio. Linda also knew that the sorrow she heard in the singer was the same sound she felt in her chest.

Her youngest child walked into the kitchen to catch Linda pulling out items from the refrigerator. The music, which had been too loud in the living room, was piercing now in the kitchen. "Mom," yelled the little boy. "Mom, Mom, Mom, Mom…"

Ivan stood up and lowered the dial on the radio. "What is it?" he asked the boy.

"Can you put on another song? I like the hot-dog song. Put it on, Mom. Put it on, and I'll dance and dance and dance."

Linda stared at the eggs, cabbage, mustard, and spinach on the countertop and then turned to the child. "No, honey. Listen to the beautiful voice, the beautiful instruments—"

"Linda," Ivan interrupted.

"Ivan, it's beautiful, I want them to experience beauty," she said, teary-eyed. She turned the volume dial.

The boy looked down and shot his hands to his ears as he ran out.

"And tell your brother to open his door," she yelled. "He needs to hear this, too."

After the boy ran out, Ivan watched her put away all the food that was on the countertop and instead pull out peanut butter and mayonnaise. "We can go out and get food," he said loud enough for her to hear. When there was no reply, "Linda—" he began.

She interrupted, "Ivan, why didn't you take care of yourself? Why didn't you stop smoking, and why did you drink so much and eat so badly? We need you."

He stared at her. The fear of dying had been enough for him to lose sleep for months, but now the fear of not being happy created an uncoordinated balance, tugging him towards bitterness. She smothered him with her emotions, and yet he was the one dying.

As the song ended, she ran to her phone, which was placed on top of the fridge—a place he hated for her to put it because, being shorter than most men, he could not reach it. Walking up to the radio, she plugged in the phone and scrolled with her fingers while nodding continuously. At the moment the nodding stopped, her pointer finger pushed the screen of the phone, creating an audible *click*.

He recognized the song as one that would play continuously from the neighbor's house, and anger filled Ivan's body. He stood up, walked to Linda, and put his chest to her shoulder. "Where in the fuck did you hear this song, Linda?"

"That's why you're sick, Ivan—you have too much anger, and it has ruined you."

Although Ivan was short and terminally ill, he was stronger than Linda. Out of rage alone, he overpowered her and shoved her hard enough that she hit the side of kitchen island and pushed it a few inches.

As the strings of Paul Cardall's "Life and Death" played, Linda stared frightfully at Ivan's nose. She was told that eye contact might prevent violence because it shows a lack of fear. Although her fear never permitted it, she had heard that eye contact could be faked by staring at the tip of a person's nose.

Ivan, who had no fear of violence with Linda, swung his right elbow into her breasts, causing her to lose a bit of breath. "You're making me jealous. What will you do when I leave? You need to leave with me."

She did not need further explanation. That sentence was all she needed to know that he did not trust her to kill herself after his death. Tears inched down her face. The sound of the strings alone could have done this, or perhaps it was the stare Ivan was giving her, the one that she had often confused for loving passion.

The reality was, though, that she had heard little playful footsteps running around the cheap linoleum upstairs, and for a brief moment, she had wondered what type of ghosts she and Ivan would become. And those footsteps, she thought, what would they sound like when her children found them?

For even in these moments of mania and depression, violence and love—the two boys had often found ways to remain outside of reality. She heard them do so as they boarded imaginary planes and got in imaginary race cars. They did so when they became invisible and when their superpowers killed the aliens. Her fondest memory was when her youngest tripped on a rug and went face-first into the tub, busting his nose and causing blood to go everywhere. The oldest, although trembling at the sight of blood, held the little one's hand and told him he was respawning with a metal face.

"Don't cry," she heard him say to his brother. "Don't cry because whatever face you're making is how you're going to stay. Look mean and tough."

The little one listened, and although they both trembled, they held each other's hands until she was able to get the blood cleaned.

It was at this moment that she wanted out of the choices Ivan had made for them. She wanted to live, but she knew Ivan, and she knew of his awareness of the proximity of his own death. And, regardless of how sweet her thoughts of the kids' laughter, imaginary dreams, dropping the children off at school, taking them to the neighborhood pool, and everything in between, she knew Ivan had not stopped staring at her. She had already stopped looking at his nose for a few moments.

"This is how it has to be if you love me, Linda."

"Could it happen while they're not here?"

"And where are they going to be? They're always here—not even their dad comes for them."

"Maybe they could—"

"Linda," he interrupted, "I feel sick, and I feel stressed, and you are not going to add more to it."

She had not noticed that his left arm had been grasping the back of her neck tightly until she felt it loosen.

"Don't hurt me," he said. "Our time is limited. Don't talk to the neighbors because it kills me. Make me feel important and loved."

She looked up towards his eyes and saw they were watery and truly afraid. She wondered how often this had happened during all the times she concentrated solely on the tip of his nose. She felt his fear of dying and his fear of feeling powerless.

Her father, while she was young, told her that men often reacted to life with a sense of victimhood, and the only true way to feel that life could be beautiful was if a beautiful woman, whom they loved, loved them. She often thought of this when Ivan seemed broken, and although she felt she had little to give him, that which he could take seemed sufficient for him.

"Can we go out once for a beautiful meal with the kids? One where they put the napkin on our laps and the waiter pushes everyone's chair in?"

Ivan smiled. "Of course, we can. We can go to a place that plays bullshit music like this, too. Because I'm sure that's what the neighbor likes to do, too."

"Ivan, please."

"All right," he said.

She pushed him back a little as she lifted up her arms to wipe the tears from her face, walked out from between him and the island, and grabbed a paper towel to clean her face. She stared at the peanut butter and mayonnaise on the counter with confusion and noticed the kitchen faucet had been running on a frozen bag of corn ears the entire time. "I'll make us sandwiches," she said and put her phone back on top of the fridge.

Before she could turn back toward the island, she felt Ivan's elbow again, this time on her back. He launched her toward the fridge, and she felt a hand on the back of her neck.

"Linda, if something happens to you, that phone should be somewhere where the kids can call for help. Don't be stupid with the things you do now."

"I'm sorry," she said, and although she wished that her genuinely regretful acknowledgment would suffice, she knew what would happen next. And as quickly as she felt a pop to her right ear and a fist against the side of her face, she faded out to the sounds of the strings and the pattering on the floor above.

Chapter 4

Multiple Sclerosis

When first diagnosed, Marco and Cate were seated in the lobby. She was holding his right hand with her left. Her right arm was extended across her chest and up towards his head, gently bringing it down against her left shoulder. She was caressing his cheek.

"What if it is something chronic?" Marco asked.

"It's not. I'm sure it's just stress," said Cate.

"Even if it's stress, that's not going away."

She continued rubbing his check and his earlobe.

"I tried to end it after our second date, you remember. I gave you an out. I hadn't been feeling well, and I had the skin cancer issue. I told you I didn't want you to follow me."

"But there I went." She laughed.

Just then, a woman in blue scrubs came out of a door. "We'll see you this way, Mr. Gamboa."

He got to his feet and took a deep breath. Cate did the same. As they walked towards the room, she held his arm close and hugged it. Cabinets, medical equipment, or other individuals, she always walked beside him and never allowed him to walk alone.

They were surprised to enter a room with the doctor already there. She was typing on her computer, but immediately looked up. "How are you both?"

"Scared," he said.

"I understand. This is a life-changing moment because now you know."

He looked up.

"Mr. Gamboa, I'll cut right to it. You have multiple sclerosis."

He looked at Cate who was looking toward the floor. "What does that mean?"

"It means that what they've thought was anxiety and stress for ten years was wrong. Now you have an answer."

"But, correct me if I'm wrong, that answer doesn't have an answer."

"What do you mean?"

"There's no cure, and I think it only gets worse."

"There is no cure, but there is a great arsenal of tools we have available to try to slow it down."

He reached for Cate's hand, and when they touched, her stare went from the floor to the doctor. She squeezed his hand.

"But, I mean, the dizziness, the weakness, the pain, the fog, the vertigo, the tingling, the burning...does that go away with medicine?"

"We hope it remits. Think of the disease as a constant progression, or as ebbs and flows with a constant progression, or even with no ebb and flow and no progression. What we do is try to keep you as normal as possible."

"What do you mean?"

"Do you remember the questionnaire you filled out before you came today?"

"Yes."

"Well, here are your results. You measured a four out of ten for each of the sixteen questions. That's what we will call our baseline."

"Baseline? So that is what I can accept as the new normal?"

"Yes, that is what we will take as the new normal, and deviations from that will be what trigger responses in medication and treatment." She handed him a paper. "This is a graph of what we show to be your progression."

He noticed that in the middle was a blue line; above it and a few inches below were red lines. "What is the space between the two red lines?"

"It's what we call WnL. Within normal limits."

"So pain, dizziness—all of it—is normal?"

"It is your normal, and the normal for many people. But we try with everything we've got to get you to stay within that range, or to lower that range to what we would think of as an average basis."

He wanted to look at Cate, but he couldn't bear to see her looking at the floor, absorbing what this meant for her. He still didn't really understand what it meant for him. "Within normal limits?" There was confusion in his voice.

"This is a lot for you to take in. I get it. Know that, where you're at, we're going to start you on an aggressive but well-tolerated treatment."

"How long will I be on medicine?"

"Well," she said as she looked directly into his eyes, "your whole life, Marco. What other questions do you have?"

"I don't even know where my ass is."

Cate chuckled.

"We have an app. Have you downloaded it?"

"Yes, it's where I filled out the questionnaire."

"Right, well, as you have questions—day, night, weekend, whenever—send us a message. Within a day or two, someone will respond."

"Okay."

"But we do have to talk about emergency situations."

He and Cate were now staring at the doctor.

From a tray hanging on the wall, the neurologist grabbed a paper that read, "Emergency Action Plan," and handed it to Marco. "If you have any new symptoms that last more than twenty-four hours, you need to call me immediately and head to the emergency room that you have selected from the app. We will already have a record ready for them. In fact, we kind of have a process where we are immediately notified if you were not able to call me."

"What happens then?"

"We pump you full of a ton of steroids, and we begin tests to see new inflammation and lesion activity. We typically will hold you for a few days until, hopefully, there is a calming of the symptoms, and we assess whether to change the disease-modifying drugs, which is what we call your medications."

"And what are the symptoms of the new drugs and the steroids?"

"Well, we don't know until we see you. There are alternate courses."

"So no one knows how bad this can get, and no one can tell me what I may need to do, or how what I do will affect me?"

"We also highly recommend you talk to a counselor, a psychiatrist. Most of our patients often benefit from antidepression and antianxiety medication. This is a lot to deal with alone, and as the chemistry in your brain changes, it can help."

"This is a lot," Cate finally said.

"Yes, it is," said the neurologist. She got up and walked to Marco and bent down to hug him. "I take this very personally, and I will help with everything I have." As she straightened herself, she asked if anyone had any other questions.

Marco stared toward the painting of a brain that was hung beside the examination bed. "Is that picture of a healthy brain or an unhealthy brain?"

"A healthy one."

"That's like putting a skinny person's picture in a Weight Watchers room."

This time, all three laughed.

"I never thought about it. One of our patients is an artist and drew it, so we hung it up. We'll talk soon," said the doctor as she walked out.

As they headed towards the hall, he and Cate continued to walk beside each other, but there was no touching until

Cate noticed the sound of a sustained drag and staccato footstep, over and over. His left leg was dragging. She grabbed his arm and walked beside him.

"Where should we go now?" she asked. "We have a full day off. Let's not go home and dwell. Let's enjoy the time."

As they turned the corner towards the exit into the lobby, they saw a man walking in alone. He had two forearm crutches. Both legs dragged, and his face was contorted. Between contorts, he smiled at them. His head shook and what sounded like just a pressured and pushed grunt was actually hello.

"Hi," said Marco.

"Hello," said Cate.

The man, Cate and Marco thought, but neither said, *Here is a timeline of what used to be and what will be.*

"I'd like to go home. I want to drink under the tree and listen to music."

"Okay," she said.

"You can go out if you want. I don't think I'll be good company."

"Maybe, but you'll be my company." She hugged his side tightly as they slowly walked towards the car.

The sky was blue, but at the moment Marco didn't notice. All he thought about was walking.

Left foot…right foot…left foot…right foot…

CHAPTER 5

Backwards Kangaroo

Penelope now made it a point to take her dad, Marco, to the grocery store a few times a week. Although he rarely left the house, he was usually never against leaving it if prompted by her or her sister.

Every time he got in the car, she'd try to guess what type of question from her father she'd get. The other day he asked her what she thought would happen if the Earth ran out of beef and water. "Sequentially, what do you think would happen?"

"Like, if there was a scarcity on the horizon?" she asked.

"No, like if one day the person who's responsible for overseeing all the beef and water just lost it, like he lost his keys or something."

"Well, first thing is…I guess they'd call HR to notify them they have to terminate someone. If it's not a well-run operation, then they might just let him know he's fired."

"Yes, that's kind of what I imagined, too. Sometimes I am afraid you aren't my daughter, but, look, we're joined by the mind."

Another instance, he asked her if she feared dying on the toilet.

"Why would I fear that? Because of how I'd be found?"

"No, because your being found would vary on the boundaries and respect your family gives you while in the restroom. There's no positive way out of this. If they come too quick, they don't care for boundaries. If they never come, then they never worried about you and already knew you took a long time."

Behind every question, she thought, he was trying to get at something larger than life. She'd sometimes ask what was really on his mind, but he often would respond, "Sometimes a turd on the living room carpet is a turd on the living room carpet, Penelope."

This time, however, he was different. He was quiet, and he seemed to not live in his head. He seemed happy to just be in the moment, and his smile almost carried an aura of stupidity. He also held her arm the whole time they drove. It was almost as if she had a childlike version of her father coming for a trip to the grocery store, a trip that might include a toy if he behaved.

"What did you eat for dinner, Dad?"

He took a few moments, looking around towards his feet and then towards her hands on the steering wheel. "You're going to laugh, but I honestly cannot remember. I did not do much today, but I feel like I did everything mentally and physically."

She chuckled and found it odd. Her father was a creature of habit. If he was hungover, he usually had potatoes, eggs, and sausage. Enough to soak up the leftover alcohol, he'd tell her. If he was not hungover, though, it was usually a protein shake that smelled like the finest cardboard from the mid-1900s. When she was little, she really thought it was cardboard and even put some into their blender one Father's Day to make him a morning shake.

By the time she parked in front of the grocery store, his childish smile had brought about a memory, triggering a childish side to her as well. When she was very little and they got to the grocery store, her dad would yell, "Quick, Penelope Jordan! Backwards Kangaroo!" And then he'd kneel, and she would run and climb on his back. They kept this up until she was well into fifth grade. It slowly subsided, starting with his bad back and then leading to him being afraid his legs would not support him, let alone both of them. Eventually, in a very somber Santa-Claus-isn't-real tone, he said he only did it because he knew it would keep her safe from crazy drivers, and it was a fun way to keep her safe—on his back instead of walking alone in the parking lot. Although she always missed the yell for the kangaroo, she never liked to see her dad say no because of something he physically could not do.

But today was different. The smile was back. The lack of radio. No singing along. Even the cold air from the darkened evening sky seemed familiar.

"Marco Gamboa! Backwards Kangaroo!"

Before she could even pause to see what his reaction would be, her father dropped to one knee and curved his back downwards as if to position himself for her to jump on.

She screamed with glee. The scream of a twenty-six-year-old woman with the heart of a nine-year-old. And although she knew better, she took off running towards her father, who remained in the position. Her father always had chubby cheeks, and every time he pretended to not smile and turned the other way, he was given away by his cheeks that further outlined his normally slender head. He was smiling—that she knew—but as she was in mid-hop, what she did not know was if he could hold her. And as she landed on his back, he raised onto his legs, and she held tight. They both screamed in delight as he took two steps before his left leg went out, and they both tumbled down and to the left. They both landed at the same time, backs facing each other.

Her eyes watered from the laughter. Her dad had carried her again. She was reminded of a quote—one day your parent puts you down and never again picks you up. Someone had told it to her dad, and perhaps that was another reason he often tried to carry her sister and her. Her sister, being younger and smaller framed, enjoyed the feeling of being carried for longer than she, but Penelope always missed it. She missed being chased, and she missed being tickled.

When her father's health deteriorated, she'd often go sit next to him on the couch and say, "Tickle me." She wouldn't run away, and he'd tickle her with his right arm as his left curled into his stomach. She eventually stopped because although he loved to play with her, it was somewhat of an odd reminder to both of them that time was passing, and it was definitely not on their side.

He rolled to his side, and she did the same as she was getting the energy to lift herself up off the asphalt. But his stare was somber. His smile, however, was still childlike. He lifted his right arm from under his body and cradled her face. "Backwards Kangaroo, my Penelope."

"Backwards Kangaroo, Dad."

She got up and helped him up. "Are you okay, Dad?"

"Yes, I am fine. Honestly, I fall worse than that more often, and that was worth it."

She now held his face. "Want to go home, Dad?"

She was sad at so many falls he had probably had when she was not there for him. She had often offered to move back, but he said he wanted her to live on her own. Not worry about him. But the truth was she always worried.

But, more so, she always missed him. There was a loneliness to him that always elicited his full attention. When his daughters asked for something, he listened. He was happy to be asked or told anything.

"No. Well not yet. I think we should get ice cream. A whole big station's worth of the stuff. We can build our own sundaes or whatever."

She smiled, and so did he. His cheeks were in her palms. And although her eyes were watery, his were now eager again. A child that evening once more.

As they walked into the grocery store and went aisle by aisle, she noticed he got things that were from what she felt was a previous life. He got pork rinds, which he hated. He got a small slice of chocolate cake. He got brownie bites. He got Dr. Pepper. He was getting all the things he hated because they reminded him of Cate.

"Dad, why are you grabbing those things," she finally asked after the Dr. Pepper. "It feels like Cate and you are hanging out." She chuckled, knowing that would never happen.

"You know what, how strange," he said. His eyesight lost in looking at things, and his mind racing to figure out why he instinctively grabbed them. The misconnection seemed to startle him a little bit.

"It's okay, Dad. Get them. Maybe you'll like them."

His smile faded for a while. He became mechanical in looking at the copy of his list, which was the same list he used every time. Again, being a creature of habit, Marco shopped for the exact same things, the exact same time of the week. He calculated what he'd use and when he'd need what. That's not to say he didn't occasionally grab something random that looked delicious, but he worked like a machine, knowing what was needed and when it was needed.

As they were in line to pay, he leaned in and said, "My leg is starting to get emotional. I better go sit over on the bench outside."

"Of course, go," she said.

By the time she got outside, Penelope noticed him focusing on his jeans, where his knee section was torn. "Are you bleeding," she asked.

"No, I don't think so," he said.

"Are you okay?"

He nodded. Held his right knee with his right arm and used his left leg to pull himself to his feet, off the bench rails. He smiled at her, but there was a sadness behind the smile he was unable to hide. The sadness was mixed in with forgetfulness, but the mixture forced him to keep what he did not want and lose what he wanted.

They walked towards the car slowly, and upon arriving at it, he used his left arm to hold the sides of the car as he made his way to the passenger side.

"I'll load the groceries. Sit down."

"Okay," he said.

The drive home was quieter. She tried to ask him a few things about stopping for food, or if any medications needed to be picked up, but he went from "No, thank you," to no response at all as he dozed off. Watching him sleep, he looked like a little kid to Penelope. She caressed his earlobes and his cheeks as he slept. Occasionally even putting her arm across his chest when she felt she was stopping a little too aggressively.

A few times, his vertigo and spasms shook him awake. When she'd glance over, on his face he'd have a look of horror that quickly subsided when he saw her driving. Hi, he'd say as he fell back asleep.

Her sister, as a child, had night terrors, and she always struggled unless their dad was around. Similarly, once she saw him, Ada would smile, say hi, and lull herself back to sleep.

When they arrived home, she gently woke him. She held his hand as she walked him to the front door. "I'll get the groceries out of the car. You go rest."

"Okay, thank you," he said with a big sigh. "Alexa, I'm home," he said as lamps were illuminated all the way to the living room.

As Penelope walked back toward the car, she heard him sit on the couch, and she heard the electrical whirl of the couch recliner kick in. By the time she walked in, he was snoring on the couch, but had not used the recliner appropriately. His torso was half hanging off the recliner section, and his legs were half on the elongated part of the couch. Although she wanted to fix him, he looked as if he was in a deep sleep.

She walked into the kitchens and said, "Alexa, turn on the kitchen lights." As the lights came on, she was a little caught off guard when she saw the same treats that had caused her to pause in the store. They were all organized on the kitchen counter. There was a paper face down with "Cate" written on it. She looked over toward the couch, where her father was still asleep. She turned the note over.

I know you guys will be hungry when you get here. I'm so glad you're home. Wake me up. I want to see you. I love you. Don't forget you girls have gymnastics and music tomorrow.

Her eyes teared up because there was confusion in his note. She and her sister had stopped gymnastics in sixth grade. Her dad was always confined by nostalgia. Could this be a note he was leaving for Cate with a playful reference to earlier times?

Penelope finished putting away the groceries and throwing away old leftovers; then she quietly went to the back porch. As she walked outside, she pulled out her cell phone and sat in a chair. She put her feet on the bonfire pit and scrolled through her contacts to find Ada. She hit Call and observed all the firewood next to the pit.

"Sup, bitch?"

Penelope laughed. "Nothing. Reading. Drinking a little. You?"

"I came to take Dad to the store."

"How is he?"

"Well, it was the nicest memory and the saddest, all at once. He played Backwards Kangaroo with me. Well, I yelled it, but he immediately crouched down. I ran and jumped on him—no clue why I did that—and we fell."

"Oh my God," Ada said amidst laughter. "Is he okay? Are you okay?"

"He fell and got scuffed up a little. He was happy, and then, all of a sudden, the lights went out for him. But what was weird was that as we shopped, he started grabbing things that weren't for him. Like, stuff I know he doesn't like. Stuff I distinctly remember Cate liking."

"That's weird. He's avoided everything about her for so long. Remember when he'd throw away her favorite cups or something?"

"Not really, it but doesn't shock me. Anyways, so I get home, and I'm thinking, *Well, maybe he's just letting go of all of that.* And I'm putting away his groceries, but everything he bought was already on the counter. My first question is have you taken him to the store?"

"No, not since a week ago. But what I'm curious about is if he grabbed the stuff then, too. I wasn't paying attention much to what he grabbed, more how he moved. There was such a carefulness to his kind of keeping his legs in check. I kept trying to make him laugh, but then the joke became him trying not to laugh."

"Well, so maybe he did grab this stuff, but it's all out on the counter, including little napkins and plates. And he had a note that said, 'I know you guys will be hungry when you get here. I'm so glad you're home. Wake me up. I want to see you. I love you. Don't forget you girls have gymnastics and music tomorrow.' Do you know if he's still talking to Cate? Not sure if you still talk to either of her kids."

"I do still talk to Rebecca, but, honestly, we never talk about them. They both became such avoidists that we, in turn, kind of to continue congruency, never brought them up. We bring up old memories of all of us, but that's it."

"I'm half tempted to hang out here and see if she shows up."

"But if the note says tonight, and the stuff is from when I shopped with him, then why would it be tonight? Why wouldn't she have already picked it up? And the gymnastics music thing sounds like it'd be a bad nostalgia thing. Dad's funny. That's not funny."

Penelope softly giggled as she recalled something. "Remember when the guy at the restaurant described the chef's special, and Dad was so into it that he told the man he was making him horny?"

Ada cackled. "Yes, that's funny. That's the shit Dad does, not fucking gymnastics."

"But there's this sadness to him now. I don't know. I know you see it."

"I do. I also feel strange when he wakes up disoriented."

"Me too."

The phone went silent as Penelope noticed a tree stump about ten feet from her. "Holy shit."

"What?"

"Holy shit, I've been sitting here talking to you and focusing on that and the insane amount of firewood Dad has that I didn't realize it. Dad cut down the tree!"

"The tree?"

"Like, the big, enormous tree we'd climb when we were kids. The tree he used to sit under and meditate. The one he'd offer beers to." Penelope was now walking around the stump. "What an enormous stump. Don't they say each ring represents a year or something? This thing has a ton of lines!"

"I don't know, Penelope. I can't believe he cut it down. Think the tree was sick or something?"

"No, no way. Oh my God, he just cut it down."

As she stood where the tree was, she realized she was now deep in the yard, and she could see into her dad's living room. He always kept the blinds and curtains open downstairs. Her dad was sleeping—half on the couch, but sleeping.

"He's like a little kid."

"He is."

"But he's always kind of been like that."

"He has, but he was still always kind of our protector. Now he bumps into everything, knocks over everything."

"And cuts down trees."

Penelope smiled. "Okay, I was just curious if Cate and Dad were talking."

"No, I don't think so. I will say this; Cate isn't well. They think she has some progressive and aggressive form of cancer. They're running more tests, but I just feel Dad would have told us if he knew. What's crazy is that now she doesn't leave the house."

"You didn't tell him? Do you think we should?"

"No and no. In a way…and maybe this is aligned with the snacks thing…in a way, I think Dad can only survive if he thinks they're coming home one day. And hearing anything else would mean what he's convinced himself is an enormous lie. I mean, honestly. And, no offense, I know you don't like to hear much about it, so I don't even tell you."

"I get it. Wow. Okay. That's a lot. Dinner Saturday?"

"Always."

"Love you."

"Love you."

Penelope closed her phone and put it in her pocket. She stepped on the stump. She wondered how much the tree had seen that Ada and she had missed about their father. How many dots could she connect if the tree told her its secrets?

She went inside, turned off the lights manually to not make a noise, and kissed her father's forehead. She locked the door and drove off.

CHAPTER 6

The Harmony in a Sorrowful Fear

The way the plane jumped into the air from takeoff felt a little different. It felt more like a jolt off the ground instead of a seamless glide into the air. The plane seemed relieved as it was pulled from the ground and into the deep, darkening blue.

For the man in 4B, however, a sensation of floating and falling began. The man looked down and saw the distancing ground covered in buildings, trees, and roads. Although the man did not think it, he already knew he would never see this place again. Even if he lived for hundreds of years, he would never want to see this skyline again.

What he did not know was that this afternoon, which was dipping into evening, would set a template and framework in his mind that caused the grey matter in his brain to fire in the most dreadful and fearful way for as long as he lived. Oddly enough, to his brain, this was the path of least resistance.

"Mr. Marco," the flight attendant said, "would you like another drink?"

"Yes, please."

As he stared out the window, he tried to imagine where she was in all the buildings, trees, and roads. He imagined her looking out of a window, wondering if that was his plane, wondering if perhaps he had not boarded to try to convince her once again. The way he pictured it, she would have been happy to have found him still on the ground. Close to her. Not being hurdled into the deep, dark blue.

Buildings, trees, and roads turned into jumbled specks. A minor drop in turbulence made him wonder if it was her, wishing he had stayed, who pulled on the plane, but anyone you'd ask would say it was just an air pocket. Although the plane was adjusting in pitch and level, his mind sporadically had the plane endlessly looping towards the ground and up again.

The sun had begun to set somewhere where the sky was now catching like fire into a sea of black. Occasionally Marco saw clouds, but the black felt like a vacuum. He closed his window shade. He did not want the gasping black to enter the plane.

"You're the love of my life. And in the thousands of years of language, that's the best I can say to beg you to stay with me..."

The thought made him close his eyes and shift in his seat. His hands were now gripping the armrests, and he could feel his pulse in his fingertips. He did not know what a normal pulse rate was, but it felt fast. How long can a heart beat fast before it gets tired?

He slid the window shade up to look again at the Colorado mountains, but all he envisioned was an image being consumed by the black as it seeped into the plane. The mountains reached for him, and the sky enveloped him. This startled him. He tightened his grip on the armrests. His pulse quickened. He could feel the throbbing in his scalp and neck.

"You're the love of my life. And in the thousands of years of language..."

The weight of the thought was tugging at him. It pulled down at his eyelids and down on his limbs. The only thing heavier was the black of the sky that now surrounded the plane as it leveled off at 36,000 feet. The nearest person to him was six rows over, and it looked as if they were asleep. He closed his eyes rapidly and felt the black of the night trickle into the plane and absorb the seats in front of him.

"You're the love of my life."

He readjusted himself again. *This sadness, this vast darkness*, he thought, *is enough to pull me into the sky, and I'll never find my way home.*

He opened his phone and looked at videos. The first was his youngest painting on a canvas and singing the Beatles' song "We All Live in a Yellow Submarine." Over and over and over, she sang without knowing the words. He opened another video, and it was his oldest dancing to the singing of the youngest, who was not in view.

"You're the love of my life. And in the thousands…"

What have I done, he thought. *I'm now six miles into the sky, no one to anchor me here, and hundreds if not thousands of miles from the ones that I'm supposed to love, and who will always love me.*

A day before, he had boarded the plane with a different confidence about Sarah. He felt then all he would have to tell her to win her over and bring her home were the stories about their time on the sofa, staring at the tree. But he knew he probably wouldn't have to say much. She wouldn't have to either. They'd just be happy to be floating in a sea of strangers. He'd play her music and listen to her say not much—just like always. He was confident she would be in seat 4A, next to his 4B.

But that was not the case.

He opened his window shade and felt his stomach drop. Although the plane stayed in perfect harmony with the sky, he was falling and floating upwards at the same time. He stared into the darkness of the sky and said quietly, "I will never see these buildings and trees and roads, and I will never see Sarah again."

Even with his eyes open, all he could picture were hauntings of his two children he had left at home while he pursued her. They loved her, but they loved him more, but instead of being content, he had abandoned them. He felt his youngest run right past his seat, but, too scared to reach out, he tightened his grip on the armrests.

"Okay, so once a week I'm going to sleep in your room. I'll take the bottom bunk. This way you get used to sleeping alone soon."

"Okay, okay, okay. That's wonderful. I'll get the room ready. I'm like an anterior decorator."

"Interior."

"Same thing, but yes. Anyways, I'll get the bottom bunk ready, and I'll put candy and..."

He closed the window shade and closed his eyes. He started trying to count the moments between the pulse beats he now felt in his throat and eyelids. *How long can my pulse stay like this?* he thought. He did not think of death, but thought of not being able to explain himself. How could he justify leaving his kids, who adored him, to chase someone who obviously did not care much for him? *What will people think if they find me in this chair, unable to defend myself?*

Instead of trying to count between pulses, he began to count the pulses with the intention of seeing how many he could count in a minute. But as the minute approached, he was too scared to open his eyes and look downwards towards his watch. Each number he counted became accented more violently through the banging on his limbs and skin. It was an orchestra building its climax by adding more instruments, more players, but it was not beautiful or purposeful. It was out of tune, making him winded, and even with his eyes closed, his eyes moved around from corner to corner, looking for something to catch him as he fell endlessly.

As he imagined the darkness continuing to force itself in and on him, Marco was pulled in every corner the black touched; his limbs were torn, and his mind stretched. And so it remained as the plane gently tilted toward the southwest, still in perfect harmony with the sky.

Chapter 7

Mom's Funeral

After the passing of Marco's paternal grandfather, Antonio, a man who rarely missed Mass on Sundays, even if he had to join via AM radio or local broadcasts on television, Marco often found solace in visiting Catholic churches. He never listened, and quite often avoided talking to anyone, but there was something in the smell of frankincense and wood. A deep, heavy wood. And while everyone went through the rituals of Mass, Marco looked around to see if Antonio's familiar face would show itself, even if only in a disappearing glance.

Although Antonio and Marco were not physically close, Antonio was always kind to him, and Marco remembered that. Antonio was organized, and Marco would often mess up his desk, Post-its everywhere, and climb atop his grandfather in any way possible to mess up his hair.

When Marco first began to experience his MS symptoms, he had a dream about his grandfather. It was in an old, familiar house, although Marco could not place it, and it was at the bottom of a three-story house with a basement that he found his grandfather. Just like in real life, Antonio had a small bed that was neatly made, next to a desk that was neatly organized. The smell of coffee filled the room, and Antonio's greeting to Marco was unmistakable.

Marco often, at that time, prayed for death. *I'm not suicidal, so I need you to do this*, he'd whisper to God.

As he heard his grandfather call for him, Marco thought it had finally happened, and he was no longer alive. He ran toward his grandfather, who was in the body of a thirty-year-old, but upon being lifted by Antonio, Marco found he was no more than a toddler.

The two proceeded to play card games on the ground, and Antonio grabbed Marco a small, kid-size cup of coffee. They watched wrestling matches on the small television located atop a little refrigerator next to the foot of the bed. When Marco got hungry, Antonio grabbed him crackers and fruit.

All was going well until Antonio's face changed. And even when Marco awakened twenty years later, he never forgot it.

"I'm sorry, son. You have to go soon."

"No, please. Don't make me go back."

"You never left, my baby boy."

"Please don't make me wake up. Please, please."

And in one of the strongest embraces Marco experienced in this life, he woke up. He sobbed for what felt like a lifetime, while his first wife and their newborn listened in the room next door, slightly drowned out by the sound of infant cartoons.

Eventually, Marco stopped finding solace in going to churches. And this was his first time in a church, although it was not a Catholic church, but rather nondenominational. He was seated toward the front, and a few pews in front of him were a giant portrait of his mother and, next to it, her opened casket.

Penelope and Ada walked to the empty chairs beside him. "How are you feeling?"

"Fine," he said.

"You don't have to talk if you don't want. I don't think anyone is expecting you to talk."

"It's fine." Marco pulled out a yellowing piece of folded paper from his interior jacket pocket. "I've kind of had this feeling this was going to happen for a really long time."

People passed by and offered condolences. At first, Marco and the girls knew who the people were, but eventually they were strangers. After a while, the ceremony began, and without Marco noticing, he began to tune out the words being spoken by the pastor. The vertigo was coming back, and all he could feel was an intensifying tingling in his legs. He began to spin and just closed his eyes. He had an arm around Ada.

"Dad," Ada whispered, "it's your turn if you want to go."

Marco opened his eyes and cleared his throat. An entire filled church was now looking in his direction. He slowly got up and walked toward the microphone. To control his equilibrium, he placed his arms on every stand and pew on his way up. Marco cleared his throat and smiled as best he could. His legs were on fire.

"It makes me happy to imagine my mom, right now, walking through those pearly gates. With Saint Peter walking her across, arm in arm, both taking slow steps for her to appreciate the sights. The family she knows and does not know, standing beside the gates, ready to greet her, ready to get to know her. I get that most of you don't believe in Saint Peter, but hear me out. It gets better.

"St. Peter right now is probably looking down at her and saying, 'Hey, wait. Your son is speaking at your funeral. Let's listen.'

"And Samantha just looked up at him with warm eyes and a smile, but inside her stomach may be feeling a little *brrrrpppp*.

"Because most of you know her as that businesswoman who went far to make sure you were happy. A lot of you knew her as a fellow Christian; she made sure you were prayed for and loved. I knew my mom as lots of things.

But as I love to laugh, my favorite was to hear her laugh. And my mother was someone who openly then secretly always laughed at a good dick joke. I'd like to share her favorite one with you now, whether you like it or not.

"For Samantha and St. Peter: Two nuns were walking on the trails within the convent walls. A couple of troublemaker kids who lived near the convent had found an old dead donkey that was fully erect, and so they cut the weiner off and threw it over the convent walls. So as the nuns were walking, they eventually came to where they found the dick. One of the nuns screamed, 'My God in heaven—they've killed Father Abel.'

"I imagine Saint Peter right now is looking a little 'Oh shit,' and I imagine Samantha is probably smiling but feeling 'Oh shit.' I imagine him telling her, 'Maybe we need to look over the paperwork just one last time.'

"When I was little, my great grandmother told me that joke. And between her, my mother, grandmother, and aunts, I was always asked to tell that joke. 'Come here, Padre Abel! Tell the joke!'

"And there went Husky Pants Marco to tell a joke he didn't understand to a bunch of cackling adults. It wasn't until I was, like, in high school that I realized the joke is about a donkey's dick looking like Father Abel's. How did that nun know that's what Father Abel's dick looked like? That's wild, right? I think it's wild.

"That was the thing about my mom. She was a certain way once she remarried, and, every once in a while, you'd see that old side of her from the corner of your eye. She devoted herself to trying to get into heaven, sometimes at the cost of who others thought her genuinely to be. And I get it. She wanted to do everything possible to one day see her mom, who, as I understood it, became a Christian right before she died.

"And that's okay. We all try, in whatever way we know how, to get whatever it is we may dream of. She once told me she loved her peace. I don't know if it was peace. She hated everyone every once in a while. Muslims, the gays, Disney. Doesn't sound like peace, but more like your local sports team. But, hey, they seem like good people. A couple of you even chuckled at the joke.

"No, but she tried. She absolutely tried to be what it took, or what she thought it took, to see her mom again. That's devotion. And I hope she finally really does have peace. I hope she really does finally see her mother, and that they genuinely have each other.

"Anyways, I will miss my mother. And I hope she's there, listening to the other dick jokes I have that I'll tell anyone who will listen. Thank you."

A few people laughed, and the majority of people clapped. Marco walked off the stage, by the pastor, and directly toward the back door. Once he exited, to the left he noticed a garden where he found an open seat on half a bench.

As he sat down, he heard the electronic voice of the pastor inside saying, "And now Samantha's business partner would like to say a few words."

"Oh shit, the whole place heard that?"

A man sitting on the other part of the bench laughed. "Yep, that was a good one."

"Thanks." Marco chuckled.

"I knew your mom."

"Ah."

"I used to be the lead pastor before I retired."

Marco nodded.

"How are you holding up?"

"I hadn't spoken to my mom in a really long time. We had a falling out."

"Yeah, she told me."

"Oh."

"Not the specifics, but I got the feeling she could never apologize, and you could never see beyond her faith."

"Something like that, I guess. I never forgave her for how she treated me when my sickness started showing. In our culture, this kind of doesn't exist. Anyways, I never forgave her, and I snapped during an episode when she started saying I felt sick because of medicine, because of allergies, because of stress. When I asked why she never believed me, she said she was just praying and praying I'd be cured. And that angered me. I was sick. I just wanted to have her sit with me."

"I'm not defending your mom. But as a parent, that's hard. There's a bit of defeat in it."

"I get that now, and I guess I got that a while ago, but we just never crossed paths again."

"That happens a lot, unfortunately."

"When I was young, we were incredibly broke. The mortgage was $1,000 per month, and she made $900. That's how broke we were. Anyways, we had stolen cable, and, regardless of what we were doing all day, we always met up in the living room during the summer nights around eleven. The cable music station, at that time, would start playing a bunch of really artsy videos, and we'd just sit there with each other. We were not only financially broke, but we were broken broke, too. Her mother had just died, and she was the foundation of her side of the family. Her and my dad had just divorced, and that was brutal. It included a fight where he threw his own mother through glass, and my mom had gone to punches with him, I think, a few times."

The pastor nodded attentively.

"Anyways, the point of all of that is that we never tried to talk about God's plan, or we never tried to figure out how to fix anything. We were all hurting, hungry, scared, but we were together. We'd get together lots of times throughout the day, but at night we'd all bring pillows and blankets to the living room, and we'd watch these videos together. Sometimes the music was so good one of us would cry. And we'd maybe hold hands or just, like I said, all cuddle up. Her, me, and my sister.

"Well, no offense, but then she remarried and became really religious. All she began to do was try to find the wrong in how she lived. Try to fix things. We became not okay with not being okay. It was almost like she wanted to take the human out of being human, being alive. And in some weird way, we just kind of lost our mom. The adventurous, funny lady became the lady who had to teach a moral to everyone.

"And, all the while, we had become addicted to just being together in silence and laughter and tears. That was gone."

The pastor listened with unparalleled attention.

"You can talk; I don't have anything else to say," said Marco.

"I'm just listening."

"Oh."

The two sat in silence for a few minutes.

"So why'd you retire? You look young and healthy."

"I retired because the closer I get to my turn, the fewer answers I have. The less I want to talk. This business is about commanding attention, being the answer for people. I don't want any of it anymore, but I understand how much our followers believe in us. And we do good for the community. But I just don't want it anymore. It's a weight I can't carry."

Marco nodded.

"Let's promise each other we'll never go to heaven," Marco joked and grabbed the pastor's hand.

The pastor laughed.

"You know, I really wouldn't like to go there. I want peace. But I never want to look at my family's face. All they did for me, and all I feel I squandered away."

"I don't think it works like that," said the pastor.

"I thought you said you didn't know."

The pastor chuckled. "Fine," he said, "if we're not dead in five years, we'll plan to never go to heaven."

"It was nice meeting you," Marco said as he stood up.

"You, too."

Chapter 8

Lost Baseballs

The kid had snuck through a crack in the fence and found his neighbor sitting at an old picnic table. "I threw my ball over the fence. Just need to get it."

"You didn't throw shit over anywhere. You're too old to be throwing balls over people's fences anyways."

The kid sat at the picnic table. "Maybe it went over two yards. We threw it really hard. I'm practicing to make the baseball team when I get to middle school."

"My friend, you're too young to be terrified. And that face on you says that you're terrified of someone. You're hiding from someone."

The boy's eyes looked in the direction of his house.

"Ah, shit's going on at home. That's all right. Look for your ball, my friend." The man finished the beer he had in his hand. And as he slowly stood up to grab another one, the boy jumped up and ran to get it for him.

"I have a question," said the boy.

"My friend, ask away if you're buying me drinks."

"Why do some people be friendly when they drink these, and others not be friendly?"

The man thought about the question. "That's why you're hiding? Looking for the ball? Because some people get different?"

The boy looked around the yard of overgrown grass and said, "You know there's snakes in grass that isn't cut."

"Probably."

"Is it Mom that doesn't stay friendly, or Mom's boyfriend that doesn't stay friendly?"

"Both, I guess—in their own ways."

"My friend, I can get this shit taken care of real quick if you want. We call the cops, and it's over."

"It's over for the cops when they leave. Not over for us."

The man was drunk, but not enough to ignore the fact that the child was likely smarter than he was because of experience alone.

"You got an old girlfriend, don't you," the boy asked the man.

The man chuckled as he tried to keep the beer down. "She ain't a girlfriend, but I think I know who you're talking about."

"Why do you got an old girlfriend?" The boy chuckled and asked, "You lonely?"

The man got up slowly and grabbed another beer. He took a pause and looked upwards towards a bright-blue sky—*A blue that never ends,* he thought. The thought made him grip the edge of the bench.

"You holding on to the bench because you're going to fall or what?"

"I'm holding on, my friend, because sometimes I think I'm going to fall upwards. I once almost got stuck up there on a flight home."

The kid laughed. "You can't fall up to the sky."

"When you're little," the man said, "you want perfection. But the older you get, you realize what you don't want is to be lonely. And you also don't want nice people to be lonely either."

"So all of you are just sitting around, being old, asking each other to not feel lonely?"

"Kind of. You worry less about it, I guess," said the man.

"I'd worry about getting Christmas lights up," said the boy. "That's important. Rumor is that Santa won't stop if there are no Christmas lights. Mom's guy says that there's a war on Christmas, and that's how you tell Santa you're a friend."

"Well, how do you wave Santa down if you're poor and don't have any lights?"

The child laughed. "I don't know. Leave the house lights on all the time?"

"I like it," said the man.

"When I'm older, I'm going to be nice to my girlfriends."

"You're going to be amazing to your girlfriends. You can also tell them as a kid you used to throw a fucking ball over three backyards away."

"Two."

"Whatever, you could throw a fucking ball, my friend. Girls love stuff like that."

Just then, a woman's voice could be heard screaming something incoherently. It was two syllables.

"Is that your name?" asked the man.

"No, but it's definitely time for me to go home."

"Come back anytime to find the ball," said the man.

"Thanks. What's your name?"

"Marco."

The kid walked back towards the break in the fence.

The man grabbed another beer and opened it. He looked up at the sky. "You pussy," he said to the sky. "You ain't fucking with me today."

Before he sat back down, he walked over to the tiny shed and opened it up. There was not much on the floor because he, before the kid had told him, knew that snakes stayed down low. Up top, he found a box with kids' stickers all over it. The box was weathered and torn at its corners. He opened it to find several balls inside. There were two tennis balls, three racquet balls, and seven baseballs.

He walked to the entrance of the shed and started throwing the balls around his yard. He looked in the direction of the neighbor's house, opposite of that of the child. The sounds of a television were coming out of an open window. He grabbed the racquet balls and threw them as hard as he could in the direction of the closed part of the window. Out of all three, only one made contact.

"Hey, what the fuck?" came a voice from inside the house, followed by the sound of a sliding patio door opening.

Marco chuckled under his breath. "Oh my God, did that hit your house? Those fucking kids two houses down have been launching shit all day. One's running around. I'll tell him to cut the shit," said Marco.

Nothing else was heard from the other house, aside from a sliding door opening and closing, then a latch. Marco sat back down and once again looked up toward the endless blue.

"If I pass out on this fucking chair," he said, still looking upward, "you better not freak me out when I wake up."

Chapter 9

Penelope

What Marco knew was that he had always loved his girls. What he found out when he saw his oldest, Penelope, breathing rapidly while trying to sleep was that there was more to love than what he already understood.

When they got to the emergency room, the real moment began. Her eyes looked toward him for comfort when the nurse pulled her small body through the triage window, but he realized he himself had no comfort in the situation and could therefore provide none.

As the doctors began yelling codes to each other, and approximately nine went into the urgent care room to begin performing tests and hypothesizing on cause of symptoms, he stayed in constant eye contact with her. He realized that true connection to her was eye to eye. She scrambled, he scrambled, and while they both were in a state of panic, he saw her eyes callous. Each moment became a moment of despair that was either a moment closer to knowing the fear that life could bring, or the isolation one might feel in their own body.

He eventually looked up at the monitor. Her heart rate was 220.

With all the commotion around, he knew she couldn't hear him. He rubbed her arm as they input in an IV. She rubbed his fingers back with the other arm.

Penelope lived, although Marco often feared a part of him had died from the fear alone of knowing that one day they would say goodbye, knowingly or unknowingly. A week later, she'd be released from the hospital.

But she at age five, he at age thirty-three—this was the day they began to say goodbye to each other.

It wasn't a thing back then for him, but it was one of the things he always remembered. When they left the hospital, it was a clear blue day. Low humidity, and there was a pleasant wind. His now ex-wife said it was a perfect day to be allowed to go home. To him, the blue felt off.

When four years later Penelope was hospitalized for the same thing, he once again took it as a nudge that he had forgotten that the goodbye continued.

Chapter 10

Letter from Sarah, 2008 [Stapled Inside Marco's Journal]

Dear Marco,

I'm sitting near the university. I'm teaching there now. There's a coffee shop that has a door inside of it that opens to a tiny bar. You should come see it for yourself. Down the street is a theater that plays old movies and for $50 will let you load any DVD you want.

I hope you and the girls are all right. Just think about it.

Love you, dude,

Sarah

Chapter 11

The Rooster

Linda shuddered a little bit when she was told she could leave work early.

When Linda came home from work, she found the air conditioner on and making cadenced sounds. It was irritating because it sounded like metal on metal, but what was more bothersome was her having to ask Ivan for help. However, she noticed the noise was loud enough to conceal her entrance. The dogs had neither barked nor run all the way to the door, and she was not even able really to hear the alarm system announce the opening of the front door.

She set her keys down and still received no attention from the animals. As she stared toward the hall, needing to adjust herself closer to the wall on the right, she could see the dogs' tails hanging over the edges of their beds. She walked closer, and, not until she was a few steps away, did the dogs look up and wag their tails at her. She bent down to pet them. The oldest, Melody, had cataracts, but she could still see recognition in her facial expressions. The youngest, Baby, was too consumed with a bone, something she assumed either Ivan had given her or she had found digging through the trash.

She stood up. The dogs continued to lie down, but looked around confusedly at something definitely out of character. Melody normally would have even gotten up to do a little circular dance around Linda, but this time laid her head back down on the side of her dog bed and deeply sighed.

Linda went back toward the entrance and took a right at the other hallway facing the bedrooms. Ivan's light was on, and the changing dimness and brightness of a smaller source of light told her that he was watching videos on his computer, but there was no sound.

"Ivan? I'm home."

There was no response by the time she got to his room, and Linda slowly leaned on the door frame from the left side of the hallway. Ivan had his two computer monitors on, each playing a different video, the sound comingled out of the speakers. He was sitting erect with his arms reaching up toward his face. From behind, it almost looked as if Ivan was in the praying posture, but a prayer he had never really been.

On the left-hand monitor, Ivan was watching a video of the kids and him playing while they were in line to get on a ride at a carnival. It was shot by Linda as the children were naming who from the family got to go on first, and whether or not all of them should be able to ride at the same time.

"Mom does make our lunches, so she should get on first, but Ivan does occasionally make them and throw in chips, candy, and no fruit or vegetables, so maybe him first."

Next to the monitor was a framed picture of Linda that Ivan had taken when they first started dating.

When Linda readjusted herself on the right side of the door frame, she realized Ivan was holding a gun in his mouth. She couldn't see Ivan's facial expression, but she could now see it was the 9 mm pistol he often kept on him. She could see his right thumb on the trigger and the left hand cupping the gun on top of his right hand.

Linda immediately gripped both sides of the door frame and stepped backwards with the utmost care not to make noise that was louder than the air conditioner. She retraced her steps toward the front of the house. She timed every step with every beat of the air conditioner. When she was at the door, she put on her shoes and looked toward the dogs. Both were asleep. She slipped on her tennis shoes quickly, grabbed her bag, and slowly opened the door.

Once she had stepped outside and closed the door, she no longer heard the air conditioner. All she heard was her heartbeat in her ears. She felt it in her throat. She stepped backwards towards the car. Similar, but not as intense, events had happened to her in the past, and she knew she had to be found in the direction toward the house or else it would look as if she was running away.

As she counted twelve steps and was in her yard, nearly adjacent to her car, out of the corner of her eye she saw something run into her peripheral, toward her back. She instinctively turned around and jumped backwards. Her heart was unable to beat faster although her body needed it. Her eyes scanned the area between the car, the yard, and herself, unable to focus fully and unable to find what she saw until she heard it—a small, muted, and meek *kakkkooeeeeeewwwwww*. She looked in confusion toward the back of her car and slowly walked toward it, contemplating, *Am I on drugs? Did someone slip me something?*

When she finally saw what caused the movement, it still took her a second to realize what it was—a tiny rooster. She didn't live in the country. She lived in the medical center of San Antonio, Texas. Roosters were things of cartoons, documentaries, and trips to someone's country home, but they were not common where she was. At best, they saw rats or were gifted rats by the neighborhood cats.

As she began to squat down towards the rooster to really verify if what she was seeing was real, she again heard the meek call of the animal. *Kakkooooeeeeewwwww.*

"The whole thing will change when his balls drop, I promise. But he's a handsome little shit. When he's older, he's gonna fuck 'em standing up. Not just lay there."

She recognized the voice. "Marco!"

Her scream startled him. "Linda?"

"Marco!" He noticed a shake in her voice.

"You okay? Sorry if he scared you. I found him wandering around. He's not really mine or nothing, but he's been keeping me company for a few hours."

Her lips trembled, and she was looking quickly between the bird, Marco, and the door. Marco was nine beers past his normal limit, but he was still tethered enough to the world to know what was happening.

Just before he said something, the door of her house opened up. He, the rooster, and Linda looked, but only Linda showed an edgy calmness.

"What are you doing home at this time and not inside with me?" asked Ivan sternly.

Marco knew enough about Ivan to know that the man's jealousy assumed that even God himself wanted to fuck his wife. "I got a rooster, and the son of a bitch ran right toward Linda."

"So an animal attacked my wife?"

"No, the rooster's balls ain't even dropped yet. I'm saying it's a baby, and it's just running around. Startled your wife, but he isn't even big enough to peck yet."

"Linda, how long have you been out here?"

"She was trying to get in, but the bird scared her, and I started to tell her a story. No biggie."

"Yeah, Ivan, I was just getting home."

Unprompted, Marco began, "I dated a real country chick when I was younger, and one of our first dates was at her godparents' house, and they had a whole ton of chickens. Anyways, it's kind of awkward because we had to go up there to check on the house while they were—"

"Get inside, Linda. I'm hungry, and your boys will be here soon, and I'm sure they're hungry."

"Bye, Marco."

"Bye, Linda and Ivan."

As they went inside, Linda seemed to wear a smile that couldn't be painted over. The smile felt forced and fearful, but inevitable.

Marco walked behind the car, where the baby rooster was standing, and started to bend down to pick it up when his left leg buckled, and down he went. Not from high enough for it to be a fall, but he had to tuck and brace for the impact. He'd have to tell the doctor about it.

He avoided hitting his head, and the first thing he saw when he opened his eyes was the rooster staring at him sideways. "You're fearless. I'm a mess, and you'll be my bluebird. I'm going to call you Hank. Hank C., if we have to be formal."

The rooster stayed in place, and Marco rolled slowly to his side, up to his knees, grabbed the bird, and then used the car to balance his final stance. As he wobbled toward his home, he held the bird close to his chest; he felt like a football player, if football players didn't run, but walked slowly and with a hobble.

"Hank, can I call you Hank? I don't really give a shit. I'm calling you Hank. Hank, that's Linda; she seems nice. That's Ivan. He'd scare the shit out of the devil if they ever met."

As he walked, Hank looked down as Marco reached the yard, staring at the sound of crunching grass. "I need your help, Hank. I tend to fall asleep sometimes, and that's okay. The fresh air is good for my lungs. The downside is that if I sleep too long, I wake up, and then I just get sucked into it. You're too young to understand it, but it's scary as all hell. I need you to wake me up."

As Marco reached his backyard, he opened the gate and put Hank down. Hank strutted around the yard and occasionally went down to pluck something off the ground.

"I wouldn't eat that, friend. But I'll get me on over to the animal store and pick you up some food."

A glass broke in the distance, muffled by the sound of brick, dry wall, insulation, and paint, but both Marco and Hank heard it. And Marco imagined what could be going on in Linda's house. Marco reached for his phone to call the cops, but he heard the kid's voice telling him it would make things worse.

Hank just kept at the plucking, and Marco put away his phone.

CHAPTER 12

Marco's Journal Entry
July 2013

When I first started having thoughts and fears of leaving the house, I attended a Buddhist Temple. I felt it was a place to try to land while I was out. It was a real hot day when I showed up, and no one was anywhere to be seen. There was some guy out back, cutting the lawn. He was short and bald, like me. I have a proclivity for trusting bald and short people. Had he also been chubby, like me, I would have trusted him with my life.

"Hi," I greeted him. "I'm new to the area"—a total fucking lie—"and I feel lost." A total truth.

"Lost like directionwise or lost spiritually?"

"Both," I half lied.

"Well, I can help with both. If you want to get back on the highway, take a left at this road, then a right at the light. Follow it about four miles, and you'll start seeing the signs to go west or east."

"Thanks. What about the other part?"

"Well, the monks are all out doing a walk, and they'd be the best to talk to, but they can sometimes be out for a few hours. There's not really, like, a plan. They just kind of like to get lost in it. A week ago, they didn't come back for over a day."

"Where are they from? This is Texas. It's hot as hell. Don't they feel sick? Do they take water and food?"

"I don't know. I don't ask. They do what they want."

There was something intriguing about not worrying about having to plan everything, but what was not intriguing was putting myself through something like that. I used to run, and the last time I ran I almost passed out from the heat.

"Listen, here's what I can do. Let me go grab a few books to get you started. I'll also get you a flyer of when the official meeting times are, and you can decide then."

"Don't grab any books. I don't have any money with me."

"Why would I charge you for books if I'm trying to help you?"

I immediately thought of when I paid $29.99 for a copy of a book on anxiety that was written by a pastor. For

$69.99, I could have had a copy which he had signed, and in which he had written a Bible verse he felt was most appropriate for my situation.

"That's great, thanks. I need help, day in and day out. I am on the verge of not only a panic attack but living in a panic attack."

"Let me hurry up and grab them."

As he took off toward a shed near the side of the main building, I looked toward the entrance of the woods where I assumed the monks had walked. I contemplated the idea of giving this man my keys, wallet, phone, and saying, "To hell with this." I would jump all into it. Perhaps my problem was that I never jumped all the way into anything. But then I thought about what the monks might think of someone just walking back there and messing up their existence.

For context, I've always had this fear of telling people—therapists mainly—my worst fears, and it messing them up. So instead of one asshole in this world who's afraid of floating up into the nothing and being stuck up there for eternity, there would be two. And like any social contagion, what if they told someone and so on? Then, like a game of telephone, what if someone added some spice to the fear, and it got real out of control? I pictured monks coming back, grabbing my keys, finding my pack of Marlboro Lights and six pack of beer I kept in the trunk on ice, and saying… I'm done trying. I'm done worrying about trying to disconnect.

"Here you go," said the man; he was suddenly beside me again. "Read through these. Start with the blue one because it gives you kind of a basic understanding of Buddhism. Then go on to the brown one because that's kind of considered the text, but if you go straight into the text, there's a lot of words you may not understand. The blue is kind of the glossary up front and context for the big meeting and conversation. But another thing to think about because all I could think about was living in a panic attack, and that sounds horrible. You live near trees?"

"I mean I have a few huge ones in my backyard. Does it matter which type of trees?"

"Nope, just any tree. Have you seen that tree in storms, hot days, windy days?"

"Yeah, of course. I'm always thinking the thing is going to tip over."

"Perfect! Okay, so next time you're feeling anxious, just keep reciting the mantra 'Powerful tree, powerful tree, powerful tree…'"

"Is it to kind of keep my mind occupied? Is that what a mantra is? Or is it to kind of live by it?"

"Well, it's both. The tree doesn't worry about what the weather is; it's just a tree. It'll always stay there, you know, especially in the safe space you create for it. Storms and weather in general are kind of just like feelings and emotions. They pass. They're not forever."

"Wow, that makes total sense. I appreciate it. I'll start these today and come back for service."

"Or don't, man. We don't care what you do. We just want you to find peace, however it is you do."

I waved goodbye and walked toward my car. I turned my car on and immediately felt the rush of cool air hit my face and wrestle with the heat and humidity that dominated the car. I opened the window to help let the hot air escape and cranked the air conditioner harder.

I looked down at my temperature gauge and saw 113. *113?! Crazy fuckers, how can you go out for a walk in this? And for days?*

But then something happened inside me. They weren't worried about it; they just did it. And I envied that; I envied it so much.

I went out the gate and took the left the guy told me to take, but when I hit a light, I took a right. I didn't even have to get to the highway. I lived about three blocks away. My short drive was mostly spent watching trees and imagining all the things the trees had witnessed. All beautiful and empty gestures combined. Intermittently, I thought how I hoped these books would help, how I could go back to that temple regularly, and how I'd tell people the story about how the man mowing the lawn saved my life.

I parked my car, got out, took a deep breath in, and closed my eyes. A dog barked in the distance, and wind chimes from the neighbors' house swung softly side to side. I opened my eyes and saw the deep dark-blue of the sky.

"Hello, my friend."

I got the feeling the sky knew I didn't see it as a friend. The blue became more menacing, and soon it'd turn into an endless dark.

CHAPTER 13

Marco, 1987, Age Four

"Mom."

"Hey, my love, what's wrong?"

"I was asleep, and I had a bad dream. I knew it was a dream, but it was still scary."

"It's okay; you're awake."

"Yeah, but I screamed at the end, and that's what woke me up."

"It's okay. Come lay between me and your sister."

"I don't want to move."

"Why?"

"My scream is what really scared me, and I still hear it."

She pulled Marco's tiny body close to hers. She patted his back slowly, and his breathing lulled her to sleep.

They fell asleep. The child safe in the mother's arms, and the mother at ease with the child in her hands.

Chapter 14

Powerful Tree

Marco was seated next to his great-uncle, who was the eldest in his family. "I'm getting divorced," Marco said.

"That's a shame, Marco, but it passes. Eventually you get over it. And I'm sure it's going to fucking hurt, but rest assured; it'll pass."

Just then, Marco's mother walked by with more coffee for the three of them.

"I'm okay," said Marco.

She poured a little into her cup and into her uncle's cup. "Martha," she said, "Martha was the one that got away from you, right, Uncle?"

As he thought about her question, the name triggered his eyes to look toward the table before he could respond. "Martha. Yes, Martha was kind, funny, and smart. And she loved me. Who knows what would have happened? When

I got the job out in Carmen, I asked her to come with me, but she said she did not want to. She said she would never find work. Had I stayed, I would have never found work."

"Do you think you two would still be together had you stayed, or if she had gone with you?" asked the mother.

He looked toward the floor and toward his hands on his lap. "Maybe for a long time, but not forever."

"Why?" she asked.

"Well, because she died while I was in the States. She died about thirty-five years ago." His face was still. His eyes no longer shifted around. "But you'll be okay, Marco. These things happen."

Marco smiled and said, "I'm glad you're here, Uncle. I've taken to walks out on the trails to try to calm my mind. Maybe you can join me."

"I'd like that," said the uncle.

"Marco thinks he's a Buddhist now, Uncle. Marco, what's that thing you say? Strong trees?"

"Powerful trees," Marco said as he looked at his uncle. "It's supposed to make you think, if the tree doesn't worry, why should I?"

"That's good; I like that," said the uncle.

Marco stood up. "I should be going. I have to get home to let the dog out. Like me, he has to go to the restroom every hour on the hour, or else the living room turns into the restroom."

Both Uncle and Mother smiled.

They hugged goodbye, and Marco walked out to his truck. He looked up toward the sky as he took the fourteen paces he'd counted between the balcony's clearing and the door handle. "You go fuck yourself right now," he said while looking up.

When he got into his truck, he pulled out his phone, unlocked it, and clicked on Contacts. He scrolled to Sam F and pressed Call.

"This is Sam."

"Sam, it's Marco. I'm sending you the money now. When can you come?"

"Would it piss you or anyone off if I'm there around 7:00 a.m.?"

"I'm going to drink enough to not even know you guys came."

"Should we check on you?"

"Not unless you're bringing breakfast."

Sam laughed. "Night, bud."

"Night, Sam."

Marco drove home. At each stoplight, he rolled the window down, put his head slightly out, and looked up. Sometimes he repeated the request for the sky to fuck itself; sometimes he just nodded silently.

He got out of his truck in the driveway and counted eleven paces. This time he did not look up, nor did he say or think a word. The counting of the paces was staccato-like. He entered the house and sat on his L-shaped couch, nearest the liquor stand. He grabbed a bottle and poured a little liquor into his cup.

He looked over toward the windows facing his yard. He looked at the tallest tree in his yard, one that stood beautifully in the distance, so that anyone inside the house could see its age by its sheer size. "Powerful tree," he said, lifting his cup toward it.

He tipped the cup back and could feel the weakness in his leg. He could feel tingling in his arm to the point it felt numb everywhere but where it tingled. He closed his right eye and looked toward the single lit lamp. His left eye showed him a dark image that looked as if the bulb was dimly lit. He switched eyes and saw it brightly lit.

"Powerful tree," he said. He tried to reach toward the stand to put his cup down, but his arm lost strength, and the cup fell to the floor. As he looked down, he tried to concentrate on the shards of glass, but his eyes were dancing in position; he tried to focus. He could feel them constantly in movement, and he closed both eyes. He could feel his eyes racing, regardless of what he told them to do.

He lay back completely and utilized his right arm to hug the upwards section of the sofa. The world was about to spin completely. *This time,* he thought, *I really am spinning off this motherfucker.*

Powerful tree, he thought. His body didn't listen, and soon neither did he. The liquor had triggered what he had now coined the "all dark." His exhaustion was that which he felt God felt when He'd finished creating the Earth. His isolation, he thought, was also similar to what God might have felt if he really did watch what happened in the place he built.

And so the all dark ensued. It was a sleep that was interrupted by spasms, feelings of falling upwards and downwards, and enough nausea to make him throw up. When he knew he couldn't hold it, he released the right side of the couch, aimed toward the floor, but his vertigo shifted the world in that direction, and down Marco went, right into what he'd thrown up. His face hit the wooden floor and glided, where it met the vomit, and skidded skin on wood. The impact did, however, succeed at one thing. It made the all dark quiet enough for him to sleep.

He woke up to sunlight coming through the windows. The feeling was foreign and startled him. He shot up off the floor and realized he had hit the sofa, carpet, and liquor table. He looked around until he saw the clock. It was ten in the morning. He got up. His leg was there, but his arm was still in another world. He cradled his chest; it often helped his arm begin to feel normal. He walked toward the backyard door. He whistled for the dog, who came slowly and achily toward the door.

At the door, he saw a paper pushed through the crack. The note read:

> *Had to go get something. Be back around*
> *2 to clean up.*

He opened the door and walked out. The tree that had stood there for over thirty-five years was now lying all over his yard in about forty pieces. Leaves were everywhere. Branches and twigs, everywhere. "Powerful tree," he said, looking toward the sky that was not hidden behind the tree, "my ass." He sat on his chair and stared at the mess everywhere. He saw birds' nests and even a few cracked eggs that had rolled out as everything came down.

"Mr. Marco!" It was his kid neighbor. "That was crazy! They were, like, crazy men, just running up and down that tree and yelling and swinging them chainsaws everywhere."

"I missed it."

"How on Earth did you miss that? They were using chainsaws and hammers and all sorts of stuff." The kid came and sat down. "Why'd you cut it down?"

"Because I ain't shit, friend. And because if I ain't shit, neither is that tree."

The kid laughed. "I mean, I guess, Mr. Marco, but, like, they're not even going to use that thing for paper or anything. I asked them. They said they just sell it for firewood. Can I steal some of it?"

"You're not stealing anything. It's my tree, not theirs. Take whatever you want, but I don't want any lip from your folks."

"All right, all right," said the kid while grabbing a few large branches and dragging them back toward the gate in the yard.

"I cut the tree down because I miss her, and because every time I miss anything, I pretend I'm the tree, but I think I'm just putting everything on that tree, behind that tree. And the tree's holding it up for me."

The boy stopped, threw down the branches, and turned back around. "What do you mean?"

"I dunno; the tree hid it. It all hurts, kid. It all hurts."

"I mean, it's your tree and all, but why cut it down?"

"Because, in reality, the tree wasn't covering or carrying shit."

The kid chuckled. "You're my friend, Mr. Marco. That was your tree, and you can do whatever you want with it. When I'm older, I want to do whatever I want, like cut my own trees down, play with my own things, and have no one bother me. Thanks for the tree branches. I'm going to make something cool and show it to you."

"Thanks, kid," said Marco, who then stood up and walked back toward the door of the house.

He walked to the sink and leaned on it. He could feel his left leg was tired and couldn't trust including it on the task of leaning. He rinsed out his mouth with warm water and washed his face. His shirt had vomit on it, so he used his right arm to reach behind his shoulders and pull it off. He threw the shirt in the trash and grabbed a cup for coffee. He hit the Brew button on the machine and sat at the kitchen table while the machine whirred, cranked, and blew steam out its sides.

He leaned his body on the table and closed his eyes. He wanted to cry. Since Cate left, he had wanted to cry, but never could. It was as if his body knew that he would not be able to handle that rush of emotion. He tried to trigger emotions by picturing her walking in right then and there, but the emotions never came. All that came was the same exhaustion as the previous night, but with nothing of the all-dark symptoms to accompany it. He closed his eyes, took a deep inhalation, and fell asleep on the table.

When he awoke, the sun had set, and the indoor lamp's timer had turned on the bulb. His stomach felt empty, and his head pounded, begging for the caffeine he never gave it that day. He stood up and felt the floor swish around him, as if he were walking on a wooden plank floating atop water.

He walked carefully toward the backyard door and opened it. His dog walked slowly inside. He looked around. The yard was empty. Not a leaf, not a twig. The nests were gone, and so were the eggs. A note atop his chair read:

> *I either envy your ability to sleep or dread your hangover. Call me if you need me to come back, but I think we got it all.*

He walked out toward the middle of his yard and looked up. It was gone. The stump had been removed, and you could only see a little bit of disruption in the ground. Thirty-five years gone.

He closed the door, grabbed his cup of coffee, and walked toward his bedroom. He sat upright on his bed and sipped his coffee. He stared at the television and waited for anything, but nothing came.

He shuffled his body to where he used to lie when she lived with him and put his back towards where she had lain. He waited for tears, but they never came. He waited to feel a kiss on his bare back, but that never came.

His head pounded, his arm tingled, and there was a feeling that there never really had been a powerful tree.

CHAPTER 15

Afternoon Naps

The footsteps on the gravel woke Marco up; he had just started by sitting on the tree stump, but was now using the tree stump as a pillow.

He looked upwards and saw his neighbor, the woman with kind eyes. She kneeled beside him and gently held the back of his neck as she lifted him into a sitting position. "How long have you been asleep out here?" asked Linda.

"I don't know. I think it was nighttime. What time is it?"

"Two in the afternoon." She lifted up a piece of paper that looked familiar to him. "I found this on your driveway. Surprised the wind didn't push it."

"Did you read it?"

"I did. I wanted to see whose it was."

He looked down toward the gravel in embarrassment.

"It's very beautiful, Marco. Here it is, so you can send it."

"That letter's been written and rewritten for years. But I never actually can send it."

"Why?"

"Because I'm afraid she'll miss me too and want to see me and ask me to do something I physically cannot."

She saw him positioning his body to stand up and reached for his hands. She pulled him up, and he noticed she tried very hard to not make a noise as his weight pulled on her arms.

"What do you mean?"

"We broke up because of my multiple sclerosis. We broke up because of the fear I had of getting sicker and how to take care of myself. I didn't let myself live, is what she said. And when I ended it, she got real pissed that I didn't try harder. She said I would have tried if my daughters had asked, but the truth is that I wouldn't have tried for anyone. I was so scared, you know? And it was either do the stuff she wanted, or possibly not be able to do the basic stuff. It's silly."

Linda didn't say anything. Her stare said she understood, and he felt warmth at her presence.

"What's funny is, when she left, I felt better. Amazing. For a couple years, and then I just got so bad. Couldn't walk. Body on fire. Mind couldn't form words. Hands couldn't type. Not all the time, but just a lot. Always fucking confused though."

She sat beside him and handed him his letter.

As he grabbed it, he looked down. "Cate always told me that, just because you write beautifully, it doesn't mean you *do* beautifully. It was how I knew to love her, I guess."

"She's been gone for fifteen years?"

"Yep, about."

"Have you ever talked?"

"No, I hid from her. Any chance I got, I'd hide. I survived by always just kind of pretending she wasn't home."

Just then from the other side of the yard, they both heard a rooster crow. She chuckled. "You kept him!?"

"I did. He's just like me; he don't work right. He does that in the afternoons, which I guess is good. Most people are already awake and at work."

"I guess that's why I never heard him do that. I'm always at work now, and I think if my husband heard it, you'd have known about it. He hates animals."

"What's funny is I don't like animals either. Don't like taking care of anyone. I'm my own animal, I suppose."

There was a pause in conversation as she smiled toward the other side of the yard, where the little rooster was walking about and plucking things from the ground. "So why not finally mail the letter before it's too late? I hear there's nothing worse than too late."

"I wouldn't know where to mail it. Honestly, wouldn't know where to email it. Wouldn't know where to text it."

"But doesn't it hurt to miss someone so much and not know if they miss you the same?"

"Not as much as it'd hurt to know they don't. And, I don't know, for me, I guess I'm just destined to miss someone all the time."

"I understand that. I miss my family, but they seem to cause more problems for us than anything. Ivan always ends up fighting with my sister, brothers, cousins—shit, everyone."

"Sorry to hear that. I don't know him much, but I feel him if he's outside while I'm outside. Like he's searching the world for problems, and it makes it just feel cold and sharp everywhere."

"Yes!"

"Do you ever wonder how we got here in life?" he asked.

"All the time. I think, as relationships fail—even little high school, puppy-love ones—we get these holes in our heart, and as we meet more people, we think they're filling the holes, but really they're just making a brand-new one."

Marco nodded in agreement. "I like that. What's hard, though, is that lots of my breakups faded over time. The last one, though, I started to only remember the good. I think it was because she was always with me when I was real sick at first, and they didn't know what I had. So we created this little covenant. So after we broke up, all I remembered was that. And then as I'm sitting there alone and sad, remembering the good, I realize that I'm starting to even forget the good. And so you just start feeling like you lost something beautiful and important, but you don't know what you lost. Turns into someone else's secret. Someone else's story."

"I think I get what you're saying, but not for me. I'm always in these fucked-up relationships, and when they're done, I just have PTSD from them, but nothing to miss of them. Everything to fear."

"Fear is awful. I'm sorry you experience that."

"We all do, I guess."

"I sometimes wonder what would have happened if I had stayed with her in Colorado."

"What? Colorado? Cate moved to Colorado?"

"No, not Cate, I'm talking about—"

Just then, the sound of Linda's patio door opened and closed. Her head shot up in instinctive dread.

"You gotta go," he said.

"I gotta go"—she smiled—"but you should really think about sending the letter before it's too late. I almost left Ivan a few years back." She was talking now in a whisper. "And although it's different than finding love, rather than trying to escape dangerous love, when the door's closed, the door's closed."

"Door for you isn't ever closed," Marco said. "You just got to ask for help."

She no longer made eye contact with him and walked toward his gated entrance. Her steps were silent—he could tell that was something she practiced.

He saw the bathroom light in her house turn on, and the sound of a plane was heard above the houses. Marco stared at the rooster. "Had I stayed with Sarah, I would have never met you, Hank."

The rooster pecked at the ground.

"No offense, bud," Marco continued, "I'd trade you for her."

Chapter 16

Juan Calderon

Juan was Marco's uncle. He had been born with special needs and in a time when the world didn't really understand special needs, and more so in a country that did not see them as something real.

Until the age of twenty-three, Juan had worked as a soda delivery man. He'd wake every morning and go to the warehouse where he and a companion would fill up a small truck with sodas. From there, they'd go up and down certain streets, delivering the soda to small convenience stores. They understood that he could only talk through broken sign language, but they knew he was reliable. Even better, they knew he did not understand money and that worked to their benefit as he made significantly less than his coworkers. But he lived with his mother, father, and eldest sister, so all he had to worry about was buying his daily pack of cigarettes and bringing home a three-liter bottle of Coca-Cola.

It was the pride of the family for him to bring home Coke. At the time, it was more expensive than Pepsi, and so it showed that even though they lived in one of the poorest and most dangerous parts of Mexico City, they were able to afford luxuries. Mind you, the family was never known as extravagant, and feeding the homeless outside even fast-food restaurants was a common practice. And not just leftovers. Juan's sister Amelia would often ask the homeless what they wanted before the family went inside, and before the family sat down to eat, she would deliver the meal to those waiting outside.

For this, and because they were part of the neighborhood, they were never messed with. The family was never permitted to intercede when a mugging took place, but their reward was to be left alone. They could leave their door open in the summer to allow for a breeze; no one would ever bother them.

But when things got worse, borders were blurred between the neighborhoods, and crime sometimes slipped into other areas. Juan was the victim of this one day when someone robbed a convenience store he was delivering to. In a city filled with violence, rape, and corruption, Juan was oblivious to crime. He lived his days delivering soda, smoking his cigarettes, and repeating his routine the next day. When he refused to get on the ground so he could continue delivering his sodas, the robbers surrounded him and beat him into oblivion.

When Juan woke weeks later in a hospital, he could no longer use half of his body, and his mind and personality became reminiscent of a child. He wet the bed every night and was mortified when he learned his work had let him go. This was before medical-leave acts, and the sodas needed delivering. It took months for him to leave the bed.

One day, Juan's sister, Amelia, was at one of the stores that had been on his route, picking up the evening groceries. The owner asked about Juan. Amelia told the owner that he refused to leave his room. "I'm unsure if it's because of the pain, because of the disability, or because he's depressed. In his mind, I wonder if he's lost his purpose."

The man did the sign of the cross over himself. "Tell Juan he can come work for me."

"Sir, he's half paralyzed. He's able to walk around with a cane, but only half his body works."

"He can keep me company. I'll pay him his pack of cigarettes for every day he comes up and keeps me company for a little while."

It took a lot of convincing because it was hard to explain to Juan what the offer was. But for the first few days, Amelia and Juan kept the owner company. Juan came home with his pack of cigarettes, and Amelia returned with her three-liter Coke.

Eventually, Juan just started to get dropped off. He'd stay with the owner by himself, and Amelia would help him home. And this became what Juan did for the man until the man died. But by then, other store owners had seen what was happening and several volunteered to do the same thing. Company for a pack of cigarettes, but the soda was off the table, even just Pepsi.

Eventually, the family had to move to a little town called Orizaba, about three hours from the city. By then, Amelia had succumbed to cancer, and it was only Juan and his mother, who was now blind. The family who received them, however, immediately went to their convenience store and explained the situation. More so, they offered to pay for the cigarettes if the owner would allow Juan to come.

"I don't want to babysit a fucking idiot," said the owner.

"Dad," said Esther, the owner's daughter, "yes, we will watch him. We'd be happy to have the company as it's just my dad and me."

And so Juan went every day. Eventually, the owner trusted Juan. Not necessarily to do anything, but he felt comfortable with his male presence and thought Juan innocuous. And as Juan and Esther began to spend time alone, something happened in Juan for the first time that he could remember. He felt something when she handed him snacks and did not let him pay for them. He felt something when she got him a cushion for his chair, and when she offered to light his cigarettes if she was lighting one, too. She often smiled at him, and always laughed with him if he made a funny gesture.

His hands were often dry and cracked, and she even opened a bottle of lotion to help try to ease what was surely now painful for him. And as the pain receded, the love Juan had for Esther grew.

At age sixty-seven, Juan did something for the first time in his life. He picked a flower on his walk to the store. When he arrived, he entered and saw the father angrily speaking to Esther and another man. Juan was confused by the way the father pointed towards Esther's stomach and grabbed the man by the neck. Juan felt scared. He did not know what was happening, but it brought up the memory of being robbed.

As Juan walked towards them, he lunged towards the unknown man to try to pin him down, but the man quickly shifted his body; Juan and his flower fell to the ground. As the father helped Juan, Esther ran into the arms of the man. She yelled at her father and kissed the man passionately. Juan felt his body ache, his strength leave, and his eyes fill with sadness.

When Juan got home that evening, he never got back out of bed. Esther never came to him the way he prayed she would each time the door opened. Regardless of how much food, water, soda, coffee, or even cigarettes were brought to him, Juan stopped taking anything in.

When the doctor was asked for help, he wrote in his notes to the family, "If the idiot doesn't want to eat, let him starve."

And so Juan passed away with a bent, dried-up flower by his bed and an unopened carton of cigarettes the father gave him the night of the incident. His body was facing the concrete wall in which there were cracks that his niece often said had been there since the earthquake of 1985.

Chapter 17

Marco's Journal Entry
The Day After the Diagnosis

I had a dream last night that I was in an apartment. I was sitting on a large, oversized single-person couch, and I had my legs up on the side like a little kid. I kept getting up and seeing a tall, blonde woman walking around the front-door area. As if she was packing her stuff. I got up on the chair and felt as if I were the size of a child. I kept calling for the lady. Kept asking her to come sit with me.

She finally did come sit with me, and I immediately said, "Please don't forget it. I could have been better; try to remember the possibility, not how I wasn't good enough. Please remember the good. Please. I already miss you." I couldn't see her face, but I knew I loved her. I stood up when she got up and tried to reach out to her, but she walked back toward the door. It was blurry, but I could see her packing and packing. "I already miss you," I yelled. "I'll always miss you."

She eventually left, and I kept calling out a name…
I don't remember what it was. The room felt darker, and
I could no longer see over the chair. I still felt her touch
from when she was next to me on the couch. I called out
her name a few more times before I heard Ada's tiny baby
voice next to me.

"Do you ever miss me, Daddy?"

"All the time."

I woke up howling and alone in bed…alone in the house.

Chapter 18

The Long Goodbye

"Dad?"

"Are you okay?" He scuffled out of bed and ran around the side, limping.

"Dad."

"Yes."

She knew this was something she had dreaded her whole life, although it was a subject rarely broached. "Dad."

"Yes."

"Dad."

"Yes."

"Dad, today is when we go outside your bubble, okay? It's Cate."

He looked out the window and up toward the sky. The sky was unseen in its blue. All that showed was the cloudiness that covered its entirety. "Yes, yes we can."

"Dad."

"Yes."

For a moment, the sky did not matter. All he felt was every sad chord he had listened to. Every sad word he had read and said.

"I will take you to her."

"Can I get dressed?"

Marco walked toward his bedroom. His left leg was weak. His left arm wasn't responsive. The world was slowly wobbling to and fro. He went into his room and pulled on an outfit—a pair of blue jeans, a buttoned-up white shirt with blue checks, and a brown belt. He put on grey socks and brown shoes. He went into his closet and pulled out a gold-and-silver Citizen watch. The watch was driven by sunlight and had been stowed away so long it was no longer telling the right time, date, or location.

He walked back to where Ada was sitting. "Do I have time to eat breakfast? How far is she?"

"Yes, you should because it's about a six-hour drive."

He walked toward the fridge and grabbed a protein shake and three beers between his fingers. He put the small shake in his front left pocket, one beer in his right pocket, and two beers in each hand. He walked toward a custom-made bottle opener that read a Charles Bukowski quote, "The fingers reach toward an unresponsive god; the fingers reach for the bottle," and popped open two beers. He turned around and took two steps. Then he stopped and turned back toward the opener and plucked it from the fridge. He put it under his arm and opened the fridge to fit two additional beers into each hand.

"I'm ready."

They got in the car. His shoelaces were untied.

"Dad, are you okay?"

"My arms and legs are on fire," he said humbly, looking directly in her eyes. "My legs are sore, my—"

"I get it. But, Dad, are you okay with what we're about to see?" Ada asked as she bent down to tie his shoes. She thought about using the story he used to show her to teach her how to tie her shoes. *"Right ear, left ear. I don't know. What rhymes? Just put one under the other one, and let's go; we're late"* was what he'd say.

"No. I always thought we'd go back," he said.

"I know. I think everyone survives by thinking we'll go back. Either to a place or a feeling."

He finished situating the five beers and started with the two opened ones. "I'm your dad. I shouldn't feel safe because of you. You should feel safe because of me."

"I'm your daughter. Nice to meet you."

He smiled. "When she left, things were bad."

"I know, Dad."

His legs became heavy. His head became heavy. The fire in the tips of fingers raged hotter. "I need to sleep."

"You sleep."

"Your sister and I recently did Backwards Kangaroo."

Ada laughed. "I heard. Heard you also broke your ass."

"Your sister ran too fast."

She smiled at him. His face was childlike. Scared. Hiding the scared behind the need to not disappoint. "Dad."

"Yes."

"Dad, we don't have to go."

His voice was lost in weakness. "But...but...if I don't... don't...I don't...if I don't..."

"I get it. You'll regret it."

His hand was atop hers on the gearshift. It squeezed in agreement.

And so they rode. Him silent. Drinking from each bottle until it was empty. Pointing to rest areas as they became available. When he was awake, her pointing to restaurants as they appeared. Occasionally he'd hold her arm as she drove. She'd hold his legs as he slept. He'd startle awake with his vertigo, and she'd wake him with her deep sighs.

When she saw the city's thirty-mile marker, she said, "Dad, we don't have to go."

Before he could respond, she realized it was she who did not want to go. She did not want to see her dad crumble any more. She also resented that he rarely left his bubble for her. He rarely left his bubble for her sister. But now he was leaving his bubble for a woman he loved and was married to a lifetime ago.

The sky was no longer cloudy. It was the blue he hated, yet Ada loved it. She was okay with all that was unknown because it was a replacement for all that she did know.

When she exited the highway, she stopped at a gas station that her GPS indicated was only 1.4 miles away from their destination.

"Dad."

"I know."

"Do you want to go to the restroom? Get a water? Anything?"

"Ada, what if she asks me why it all went bad? What do I say? Do I say it was because of me? Do I say it was because of her? Do I tell her why I avoided her? That it was too much for me to see her face? Do I tell her that she's a ghost that haunts me even on this ride? Do I tell her I avoided everything that reminded me of her? Do I tell her I still love her? Do I tell her?"

"Dad."

"Yes."

She wanted to tell him that she was no longer there. That it was really just a formality, that a few people were able to visit her before life support was pulled. But she did not have the heart to tell him that what he so obviously was waiting to do was no longer a possibility.

He continued, "Do I tell her?"

"Let's just get there. It'll come to both of you." She hated her lies, but realized now that she was only doing what he had done her whole life when things were too scary or too sad.

He squeezed her hand on the gearshift. "This is probably stupid for all of us. Love has been broken since we could write. Since we could tell stories. But it's one thing to read it, and another to live it. It's also another thing to know you've lost it twice and been unable to take it."

"Twice?"

He began coughing. She looked at him to see if he needed help, only to realize he had opened the two remaining beers and was drinking them as they pulled up the cement driveway toward the hospital's parking garage.

When she parked, he said, "Ada."

"Yes."

"When we divorced, you were so hurt. You never responded to her; I don't know if you were hurt, or if you were protective of me."

"You were my hero. And she hurt you. Even today, I feel stupid driving you here."

"I understand. Have I told you about Juan?"

"Dad, Cate's in room 324 on the third floor. I will wait here. I want you to enjoy it, but I've been told her family will arrive later; you should leave before they get here. Everyone wants a turn at what you're getting."

He bent down slowly and kissed her hand on the gearshift. Then he got out of the car and made sure his shirt was tucked in. He reached into the rear seat, pulled out cologne, and sprayed himself. As he felt the weakness in his left hand, he noticed the wrinkles in his hand that stretched up his arms, through his tattoos, and into his shirt.

He walked toward the walkway that connected the garage to the hospital. He looked above and saw the blue of the sky. And although he wanted to stop and scream at all he feared, he walked toward an old, dying love.

The parking-garage walkway connected to level two of the hospital. The garage was toward the left, and he got to the third floor in just a few moments' worth of thoughts.

On their third date, they had met at an Italian restaurant. It was not a cozy one. It was one frequented by all the executives with whom he was friends. It was a restaurant in which you behaved, but Cate and he had spent the entire time kissing. Before the meal was ordered, his face was covered with her lipstick, and the waiter smiled because it was uncommon for thirty-year-olds to make out in public. It was hope.

He thought of the first time they slept together in a new house, and she told him she loved him. "I love you, too," he'd said.

"No, don't be a copycat. I love you, and you don't know what that is."

The memory triggered a smile as he walked to her room…which was exactly when he realized the gravity of the situation. Thirty years later and he was still in love, but he'd never been happy since they parted. He'd never again be a thirty-year-old with lipstick all over his face in a business-district Italian restaurant.

As the bell rang and the elevator doors opened up, a nurse at a station smiled at him. "Room 324," he said.

She smiled in recognition. She knew he was coming; she had been told memories by the family. "This way."

He noticed that as he walked, the hallway began to shift. His steps seemed twisted, and the tunnel vision made all the squares in the floor morph into rectangles and squiggly lines. His left eye only saw shadows, and his feet and now arms were on fire.

"You're Marco?"

He nodded.

"The family said she called you Grumpy."

"She did," he said.

"They said you made her laugh all the time. And that you liked to hump her leg."

He laughed and began to cry, all at once. "I did. It was how I knew how to play with her. How to make her laugh."

"Well, Mr. Marco, she remembered until she didn't."

They were at her room. Rebecca stood from the chair beside the bed and walked toward him. The nurse gave her his arm and said, "I think his side is weak."

"Hi," said Cate's daughter, Rebecca. She helped him walk to the side of the bed.

Marco found a small, frail body under the sheets. He saw dark hair down to the shoulders with sporadic spots of scalp showing. He took a deep breath. "Can she hear me?"

"I don't know. But I'll leave you until my dad, aunts, and cousins come."

"Okay."

As she walked out, she slid the door closed.

"Cate?" It had been ages since he had heard his voice call her name.

She was silent. The body lifeless. Monitors beeped, and air vents whirred. Her back was to him.

He lunged toward the bed. His face was planted against the bed as his legs worked to push him upwards. He touched her back and only felt bones. He pushed his face against her back—covered in gown, sheets, and blanket—and kissed her back. He put his face back down against her skin and began to cry. Finding strength, he used his left arm and pulled the coverings from her shoulders and exposed her gown. As he used his left hand to open her gown, his right leg and right arm found the strength to push him upwards toward her exposed back. He kissed her.

In case she hadn't felt it, he loudly plucked his lips and made a pucker sound. He remembered decades before when he was waking up to pee seven times a night at the early onset of his disease. Every time, she looked up and blew him a kiss. She never became angry at his waking her.

His legs both worked in conjunction to propel him so that he was able to roll onto her bed. He could see her back more clearly. Her moles scattered across her back.

"My little flour tortilla." He chuckled. He cried. His head got heavy.

All that he wanted to tell her could only now be told to a room of machines and tools. She was gone.

He slowly shifted her so that she was lying on her back. He put his head on her pelvis and looked upwards at her, now seeing her face. A face different by time's standards, but identical to the one she wore the night she left, sans the anger.

"Every time we fought and made up, you'd ask me to lay completely on you. I must have outweighed you by a hundred pounds, but you always asked for that. You said it was your favorite."

For the moment, the best he could do was to keep his head on her pelvis. He placed her left hand atop his left hand, and held both with his right. "Please wake up. I have so much to tell you. So much I missed."

The beeps were all that responded.

"Please come back."

Beeps and whirring.

"I was meant to miss everyone, but I wasn't equipped to miss you."

As he grew accustomed to the beeps, he hoped only for a squeeze. A movement. A glimpse of her eyes. But all he got was a heaviness in his head that afforded him a final opportunity to fall asleep next to her. He climbed now beside her and rolled her back onto her side. He put his right arm under her head. And before he put his left arm on her waist, he raised her left arm up towards his face, her hand behind his head as if she were pulling his head towards her. Once he situated his head next to hers, he placed his arm around her.

"I'd like to go now too, if that's okay, Cate," he said aloud.

And for what felt like the first time in forty years, he slept without any symptoms. He slept. He was not sure for how long, but before he knew it, a nurse was smiling at him as he was being buckled back into the car with Ada.

He began to cry as he saw her face. "I want to go home," he said.

She nodded.

"Is she gone?"

But before she could respond, the burning in his entire body took over, and he was deep in a dizzying and burning sleep.

CHAPTER 19

Christmas Lights

After losing Cate and his mother, Marco had taken to writing his mother letters. "I'd rather miss you and love you, than have you and hate you," wrote Marco, trying to explain his absence to her while she was alive.

He was interrupted by the steps of a man carrying a camera and tripod. The man saw Marco sitting on his porch and stopped in front of him.

"Did you know the lady a few houses down?"

Immediately, Marco thought of the boy. "A little."

"Murder-suicide. Kids inside waited to do anything until the sun was up. Didn't even go into the room because they knew. Called their sister in the morning, and she came and discovered both bodies and the two boys in their room. Both their pajamas were wet with piss because they didn't want to go into the room.

"So how well did you know them?"

"Not enough," said Marco.

"You just said you knew them a little."

"Yes, but not enough to talk about them to anyone."

Marco grabbed his rooster's ashes that were now in a Pepsi bottle, and his dog's ashes that were now in a Marlboro box. He went inside. He could hear the boy's little voice echoing in his mind. The boy's voice asking him questions, and Marco's voice answering the questions. He sat on the couch and looked at the picnic table where they often sat to talk.

Marco felt dread, and so he pictured his own mother patting his back during a nightmare when Marco was little.

Marco pictured the boy.

Marco pictured Ivan and Linda.

Marco pictured the boy.

Marco woke up a few hours later. It was still the same day. The sunlight stank the same way. He stood up and grabbed the phone out of his pocket.

"Penelope texted," he said to the Pepsi bottle and Marlboro box. "She's going to take us to the grocery store," he said, looking at his phone and watch, "in thirty minutes."

He limped to his room. His left leg was gone, and most of his body rested on his right leg during all steps. As he got to his room on the second floor and looked out the windows that overlooked the pool and backyard, he saw dog toys he never threw away and a chicken coup that never housed any chickens, but for a time just one rooster.

"Duke, I'll get you some chicken to boil. Hank, I'll get you some corn," he said to the bottle and the box.

He looked at the bed that he only utilized half of; the other half never came undone. He sat there in silence. He never changed until the honking of the horn at the front of the house snapped him out of his trance.

He slowly went out of the room and down the steps. He put the bottle and the box on the floor near the front door. "I'll be back."

He closed his door and saw Penelope in the driver's seat of the car parked in his parking lot. He twerked in front of the car, holding on dearly to his cane, and then threw up a gang sign. He saw her smile as he walked to the passenger door.

"Hi, my love."

"Hi, Dad."

"How was your day?"

"It was good, but what's with all the news-station vans down the road?"

Marco clenched his right hand and tried to do it on the left, but nothing happened. "I don't know. I've been sleeping all day."

Penelope pulled the car down the driveway. She turned the wheel to the left and then drove onto the street, towards the exit of the neighborhood. As they drove down the street, Marco saw the news-station vans. But that's not what hit him.

As the car approached the house, he saw that the Christmas lights were on. As he followed the strands of Christmas lights, he saw that they were plugged into a wall socket without any timer or smart sensor.

"He asked for them to be turned on."

"What?" said Penelope.

"When he got picked up, he asked for his family's lights to be turned on."

Penelope parked next to the vans in the middle of the street and looked toward the house. The car hummed in Idle. "You knew the boys, didn't you?"

"Just one." Marco sighed. "The other was always in his room, playing video games. But the oldest would often find me outside, passed out or in the middle of fighting the sky's blue," he said and then paused. "And he knew something was wrong, so he'd just talk to me."

"Dad, have you called the family to see if they're okay?"

"No."

"Dad, but—" Penelope stopped as the Christmas lights made her stomach turn.

"It was a murder-suicide."

"How do you know?"

"The newspeople told me earlier."

"Did you—"

"I remember taking you shooting when you were little. You couldn't have been more than five and your sister maybe three or four. I took you for hot dogs before then."

"Mom has a picture of that. We all have on huge earphones for the noise."

"Even with the noise-canceling earphones, you two flinched. And you were having a good time, but you flinched. And I remember thinking, what if in life you heard the gunshot without earphones? What would you do?"

Penelope grabbed his hand.

They both looked up at the lights, but he began to sob. "Your little hands trembled when I had you guys hold the gun, and we shot together."

She held his hand tighter. The lights seemed to glow braver. "Dad."

He quieted.

They sat as the car hummed and the radio lightly played notes only a dog could hear at this volume. They both looked up toward the top pitch of the house, the highest place the lights were stapled to the corners.

"But did he put them on to show where he needed help? Or did he put them on to show he was okay?" he asked through tears.

She held his hand. Both sat in silence until a news van that was coming in from the street honked for them to move.

"Regardless," she said, "they're up, and we get to see them."

CHAPTER 20

Colorado 2009

The plane broke through the clouds, and Marco could see the range of mountains surrounding the city. The sky was a magnificent blue that, to Marco, signified anything was possible. All he saw were the smiles of the two passengers seated on the aisle to his left. They were celebrating, and soon, he thought, he would be too. On a flight back home with Sarah. He in 4B, and she in 4A. They'd have a drink. He'd have a Shiner Bock, and she'd have a dirty gin martini.

When he landed, he used the escalator in the airport and descended to a mostly empty lobby. Below him were a few men in black suits, each holding up a sign bearing someone's last name. One read Gamboa.

Marco greeted the man holding the sign and said, "I'm Marco."

"Hi, I'm here to take you to your car."

"Okay, thank you."

Marco held out a bag for the man to hold, but the man smiled, turned around, and walked toward an exit. Marco followed. They walked toward general exits, and Marco continued after him.

Drivers in the past were more talkative and always carried bags. They'd often walked side by side. They also always called Marco by his last name.

They continued through exit doors, and as Marco struggled to keep up, he was tackled from the right. It was Sarah.

"BAAAAAAHHAHAHAHAHAHAHAHAH."

He smiled; her laugh alone would make whatever situation perfect.

"What?!"

She kissed him. Quickly, profusely, and fast enough to explain in small bursts that she paid some stranger to hold up the back of an Airport COVID sign they had found on the floor. The back of the sign now read Marco.

He hugged and kissed her. A cop came by and told them they needed to get out of the area, but they never heard him. In their own world, at their own time, they slowly picked themselves up and held each other for as long as they could. Eventually, the world began to spin, and in the movement of the spin, they walked toward her car, parked about a hundred yards away in a parking garage.

She drove and talked to him. She not only told him of her life, but she told him about the city—more importantly, what he would love about the city. What Penelope and Ada would love about the city. Some of the things she said to describe activities were, "It's magnificent, because...," "It's perfect how...," and "It's important to them because..."

Marco could not listen to the rest. He was primarily focused on her mouth and eyes as she described something she had been experiencing since she got here. It weighed on him that he had never considered coming here to stay. It had never occurred to him having to tell Penelope and Ada that they had to leave their homes and few family members. It never occurred to him that the decision was his or Sarah's. And in a way, not hers and not his. They both had made a decision that perhaps was mentioned to each other, but never truly absorbed.

They sat through lunch in a small café with a bottle of wine. She listened to his stories. His clumsiness was bothering him; he also sometimes slurred; he thought it was due to his health. Twice, he was warned about strokes, but the scans, not MRIs, ordered showed nothing.

She said she'd call his doctor's office next week. "I'm friends with some of the staff there from rotations. Maybe I can see if they can tell me more."

It was not until bed that evening, after having had each other, that they were lying together and Sarah asked him,

"You will come, won't you? I have a place, job, resources, schools—everything we need here."

Marco listened and thought a long time. It was not until he heard her steady breathing, indicating sleep, that he said, "I don't know. I cannot leave my girls."

She opened her eyes. "You're not leaving your girls. You're bringing them."

"I'm working on my book. I have a job that pays well and lives the girls smile about."

"All of that could be here. With mountains to watch you guys."

He smiled. "But I have everything for you. I have money, so you don't have to worry how long it takes to get into medical school at home. I've got enough room in the house to make it yours. And we have…well, everything."

"But maybe everything we have there is not everything we need…I need."

He looked down, and her eyes followed. They shared a promise that was always kept. Whenever there was disagreement, they'd pause the debate or conversation. They'd accept what the other wanted and choose whether to stay or leave.

Both remained at peace as they held each other. He fell asleep first, but not deep enough to not feel her soft kiss on his forehead before he cradled deep in her embrace and his dreams.

He missed that she said, "Thank you for believing in me," as he slept.

She missed that he said, "I'm sorry," as he got up quietly in the morning and began to pack his bags.

She missed that he said, "I know something is wrong. And I know I will be a burden. And I know you would watch me, love me, and fill me with joy, but I would only do that if I could reciprocate." At this point he whispered, "But I don't want that to be deadweight only for you. Even without being able to tell you or show you, I would hate the look you gave me as I fell deeper into a puddle of endless blue—too deep to see you or the girls."

After he said that, he realized he was lying. He wanted to be sick at home; he was too scared to be sick anywhere else. And as he acknowledged his lie, the room began to feel too big. As he walked closer to the door, he heard her voice.

"Please stay."

He turned and ran toward her. He dropped what little he had in his hands and jumped atop her in a way to avoid crushing her. He kissed her, and their tears fell slowly to their open and connected mouths.

She knew, and he knew.

"You're limping. There's more happening that I don't know. I figured you'd eventually say something. You're the love of my life. And in the thousands of years of language, that's the best I can say to beg you to stay with me. I'll protect you. I'll learn so I can care for you."

He got up. Cried and wailed for a second with a resounding howl of grief.

She hid most of her face under the covers.

He opened and closed the door without allowing for pause. He closed it softly, but with enough vibration to cause the two backpacks she had purchased—with the initials *P* and *A*—to fall off the stand where she had put them.

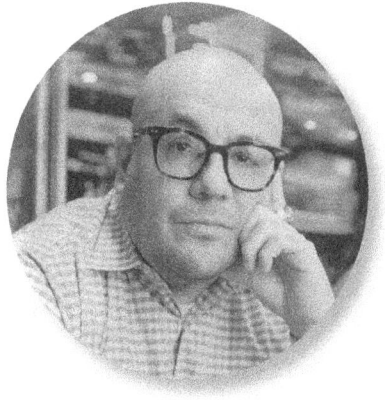

Let's Connect

Find out more about Marco Antonio Gamboa
at the following links!

Facebook: WnLmarco

Instagram: @wnlmarco

*9 7 8 1 6 3 7 6 5 4 9 5 8 *